EAT | MOVE | PERFORM

VOLUME 1 – NUTRITION & SUPPLEMENTS

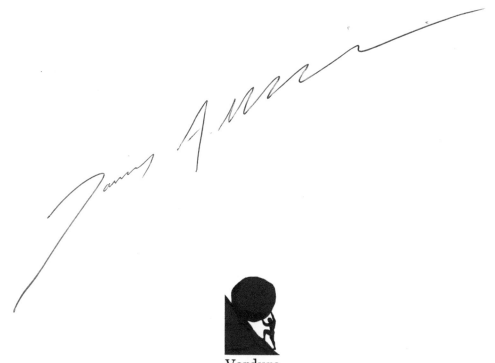

Verdure
Mettle

James A. Hickman MSc, CSCS, CISSN

This book is copyright © by James A. Hickman
First published in 2020 by Verdure Mettle Publishing
Office 41765, PO Box 6945, London, W1A 6US, United Kingdom

Written by James A. Hickman
Edited by Emma Lewis
Cover & Interior Design by James A. Hickman

ISBN: **978-1-8381357-0-6 (Paperback)**
ISBN: **978-1-8381357-1-3 (eBook)**

British Library Cataloging in Publication Data
A catalogue record of this book is available from the British Library

CONTENTS

Volume 1 - Nutrition & Supplements

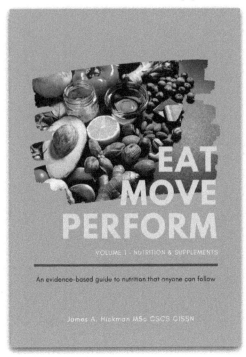

Energy Balance & Metabolism

Macronutrients

Micronutrients & Hydration

Meal Frequency & Timing

Bioavailability

The Gut Microbiome

Diets

Supplements

Volume 2 - Exercise & Performance

Core Strength & Stability

Mobility & Flexibility

Endurance

Hypertrophy (Muscle Growth)

Strength & Power

Speed & Agility

Rest & Recovery

Periodisation

Exercise Technique

Movement Screening

Sports Psychology

Performance Testing

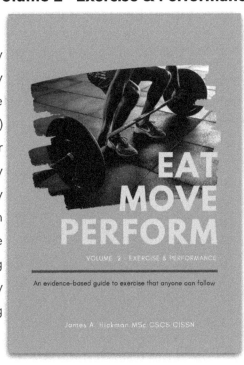

ABOUT THE AUTHOR

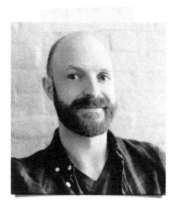

James A. Hickman is a Sports Nutritionist, Exercise Physiologist, and Strength & Conditioning Coach with many years of experience in helping people to improve their health and performance. James often receives praise from his clients and colleagues about his ability to communicate with anyone in a language that is understandable but rich with detail. James began his interest in sport science and nutrition at a young age while being recruited to play college basketball in the USA. This passion to improve his performance developed into a desire to help others achieve their goals and into a career in facilitating behaviour change.

James studied Human Biosciences at the University of Plymouth and Sport and Health Sciences at the University of Exeter. While working as an Exercise Physiologist, James completed a professional diploma in Health and Well-being Physiology, became certified as a Strength and Conditioning Coach with the National Strength and Conditioning Association (NSCA), and certified as a Sports Nutritionist with the International Society of Sports Nutrition (ISSN). James is an Accredited Anti-Doping Advisor for UK Anti-Doping (UKAD) and has previously worked as an Expert Panel Reviewer for the British Association of Sport and Exercise Sciences (BASES).

As a healthcare professional and performance specialist, James can critically analyse all of the available scientific information on nutrition, supplements, exercise, and performance and deliver clear evidence-based guidance that everyone can follow to achieve their goals. James' passion to help others is evident in his writing, through his careful attention to detail and desire for everyone to have access to the best advice and guidance. James spends the majority of his free time with his wife Lucy in London where they enjoy exploring the city and trying new cuisines. James is an avid reader and learner, having taught himself to speak conversational Spanish and to play the guitar. James is now retired from coaching and playing basketball but still stays active through gym-based training, swimming, and running.

PREFACE

The amount of available information on nutrition, exercise, performance, and health has never been greater, yet most people still struggle to tell the difference between scientifically accurate and helpful information and the latest pseudoscience diet fad or exercise trend. So, what is the best option for your health and performance? Should you follow a Vegan diet or a Carnivore diet? Should you focus on Powerlifting or are Ultramarathons the best for longevity? Does intermittent fasting hold the cure to the obesity crisis or is eating every 2 hours the answer? The amount of conflicting information in the media is overwhelming and can leave you feeling paralysed from fear of making the wrong choice.

What is so desperately needed is a book providing the pros and cons of everything nutrition and exercise-related and giving unbiased, evidence-based guidance on how to eat right, move well, and perform at your best. Now I have read a lot of books on this subject and try as I might, I couldn't find one I'd recommend to the average reader because you either have fantastic textbooks with the best possible information but aimed at students and academics, or popular media books which are often very inaccurate and provide little to no balance to their arguments. I therefore decided to write the *EAT* | *MOVE* | *PERFORM* book series drawing upon my experience as a sports nutritionist and strength and conditioning coach, and trawling through every useful piece of research I could get my hands on along the way.

The *EAT* | *MOVE* | *PERFORM* book series is divided into 2 parts. **Volume 1 - Nutrition & Supplements** covers key topics including energy balance, metabolism, macro-/micronutrients, hydration, nutrient bioavailability, the gut microbiome, meal frequency/timing, diets, and supplementation. **Volume 2 – Exercise & Performance** covers mobility/flexibility techniques, core strength conditioning, hypertrophy, power, endurance, speed, and agility training, periodisation of training plans, optimising recovery, performance testing and more. Wherever possible the language throughout has been kept to a detailed but easy-to-read style, explaining any technical terms where necessary and references for all sources provided for the more studious readers. Each chapter also includes a "Practical Applications" section, to show you how to apply the information in a useful and bespoke way to meet your health and performance needs.

This book series has been a labour of love and I hope you can find the answers you are looking for to empower you to design your own nutrition and exercise plans and achieve your goals. This project would not have been possible without the love and support from my amazing parents, dear friends and loving wife. None of this could be possible without your support too so thank you for your purchase and I wish you the very best for the future.

Nutrition & Supplements

INTRODUCTION

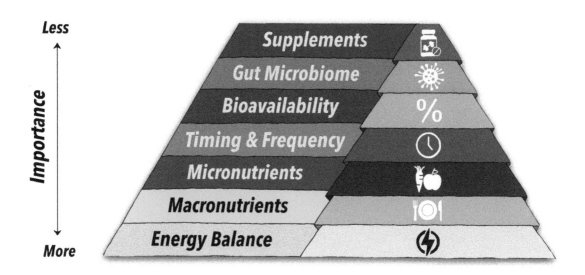

When learning about nutrition and supplementation it is important to understand the relative importance each aspect has on your overall health and performance. To accomplish this we often use nutritional pyramids (like the one above) to represent the most important foundations of a good diet at the bottom and the less important factors at the top.

The base of the pyramid and the foundation of an effective nutrition plan is *Energy Balance*, which is covered in Chapter 1. If your energy balance is not in line with your goals you will struggle to make any discernible improvements even if modifying the higher areas of the pyramid. The next level is *Macronutrients* which are covered in Chapter 2. Macronutrients are where you get your energy and building blocks to build a strong and healthy you. Carrying on up the pyramid we have *Micronutrients* which are covered in Chapter 3. Micronutrients are all the little extra bits that help to fight disease and keep everything running as it should. *Meal Timing & Frequency* which is covered in Chapter 4 is the next level and acts as the transition between the factors which have a significant impact on your health and performance and the areas which have a much smaller effect. Timing and frequency are all about how many meals/snacks you eat a day and what time you eat them. Next up is *Bioavailability* and *The Gut Microbiome* which are covered in Chapters 5 and 6 respectively. Bioavailability is about how much of your food you can utilise and the gut microbiome is how the colony of microorganisms within your gut can help you to stay healthy. The top of the pyramid is *Supplements* which is covered in Chapter 8. When all the preceding factors are optimised this factor has the smallest effect and you may not even need to use any supplements to stay healthy and reach your goals. Supplements can include anything from multi-vitamins to anabolic steroids that are used to boost your health and/or performance. Not included on the pyramid are *Diets* which are covered in Chapter 7. Diets do not appear on the pyramid as there is no one specific diet that is necessarily perfect for everyone.

Nutrition pyramids should never have a peak, as our knowledge and understanding of nutrition and supplementation is unfinished and you should always be open to learning and adapting your practices to meet the most up-to-date and scientifically valid guidance available.

1

ENERGY BALANCE & METABOLISM

How much do I need to eat and is what I eat important?

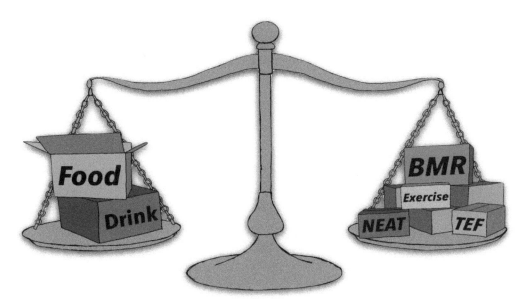

Energy balance is defined as *the balance between the calories you consume each day through food and drink, and the number of calories you expend through physical activity and your body's normal physiological processes.* This principle can be stated even simpler by the phrase *Calories In vs Calories Out (CICO).* However, problems arise with understanding how surprisingly complex this balance is and how it is not a fixed value. The human body is constantly trying to keep a careful equilibrium between the building and breakdown of every cell in your body. To do this, you must eat enough calories per day including several essential nutrients from your diet to account for the energy lost from just keeping your body functioning normally. When you start expending more energy by exercising or start ingesting too much energy through excess food and drink, the balance between your calories in and your calories out are no longer in equilibrium and changes in your body composition occur (i.e. you will lose or gain weight). To understand why this equilibrium is so complex you first need to understand the four components that comprise the calories out side of the calories in vs calories out equation. These four components are known as your *Total Daily Energy Expenditure (TDEE).*

Total Daily Energy Expenditure (TDEE)

The four components of your total daily energy expenditure are your Basal Metabolic Rate (BMR), Non-Exercise Activity Thermogenesis (NEAT), The Thermic Effect of Food (TEF), and Exercise Activity (EA). Each component has a varying contribution to your TDEE dependent upon whether you are in a caloric deficit or surplus, the amount of activity you are engaged in, and the types of food you eat.

Basal Metabolic Rate (BMR)

BMR is the largest component of your TDEE, making up approximately 60 - 70% (however, this percentage may be lower in very active individuals). BMR is the minimum amount of energy needed to sustain life and accounts for all the energy that is required to run your basic bodily functions including, pumping blood around your body, creating hormones, thinking, breathing, etc. BMR can be measured using a Metabolic Cart

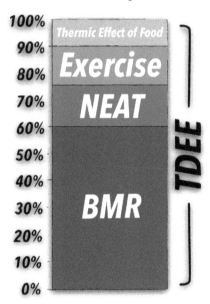

after a 12-hour fast while resting and in a neutral temperature environment. However, for most people predicted BMR calculations (covered later in this chapter) are used as a cheaper and more convenient alternative for determining BMR. Your BMR is largely determined by how much lean mass you have (i.e. muscle) and how efficient your body has become at obtaining needed energy from your food. Overweight people are more efficient at obtaining energy from food and as a result store greater amounts of excess energy as body fat. Lean people are much more wasteful and therefore do not store as much body fat due to a less efficient ability to obtain needed energy from their food. However, during periods of caloric restriction your body will become more efficient at obtaining energy from your diet and your BMR will reduce as a result[1].

Non-Exercise Activity Thermogenesis (NEAT)

NEAT is the second-largest component of your TDEE, making up approximately 15% in sedentary individuals and as much as 50% or more in highly active individuals. NEAT accounts for all the involuntary movements you make each day like using your devices, fidgeting, talking, moving around, etc. NEAT can decrease significantly when you become more active as you unconsciously move less in your day-to-day activities to compensate for the energy you are expending by engaging in more structured exercise. It is therefore recommended to include goals for staying active during your day, as well as exercise goals when trying to lose weight to help attenuate this effect.

Thermic Effect of Food (TEF)

This component accounts for the energy used to ingest, metabolise, absorb, and store energy from your food and makes up approximately 8 - 15% of your TDEE. The process for storing fat is very efficient and as a result, has the lowest TEF (0 - 3%). Carbohydrates and protein require more energy to convert surplus energy into body fat and as a result have a higher TEF (Carbs: 5 - 10%, Protein 20 - 30%). In theory, 3 months of 400 excess calories of fat or carbs vs 400 excess calories of protein could result in a greater effect on weight gain. However, this component of your TDEE remains relatively stable, unless in a caloric deficit where it may reduce slightly. Eating a high protein diet may help to attenuate this effect and also aid in satiety (i.e. feeling fuller), which could result in better diet adherence[2].

Exercise Activity (EA)

This component is what is referred to when generic government advice says "move more" and only accounts for 15% of the average adult's TDEE and as much as 30% of active individuals. You can see why the phrase "eat less, move more" doesn't cover the complexity of the calories in vs calories out equation and causes confusion. Despite this relatively small contribution to your TDEE, exercise activity is still the component you have the greatest influence upon and increasing your exercise levels will have a significant effect on the number of calories you expend. The amount of energy expended during exercise (i.e. calories burned), is determined by the duration and intensity of the activity performed. The effect exercise has on your TDEE is known as metabolic cost and is measured in *Metabolic Equivalents (METs)*, which represents multiples of your BMR. Resting is equal to 1 MET and all exercise costs more METs. For example, strength training equals 6.0 METs, meaning you will burn 6 fold the number of calories while engaged in strength training exercise compared to resting[3]. To help you understand how to calculate your TDEE we will use two hypothetical example individuals with varying body composition and activity levels. These will be Mr Couch-Potato and Miss Gym-Bunny.

Mr Couch-Potato.   **Miss Gym-Bunny**

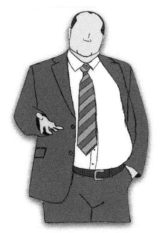

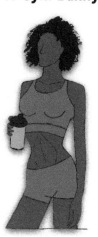

41	Age	24
178 cm	Height	162 cm
93 kg	Weight	55 kg
34%	Body Fat	21%
Desk-based job and no exercise	Activity	Active job plus gym training 4 days/week

3

BMR Calculations

TDEE calculators work by first trying to estimate your BMR using key variables such as weight, age, sex etc., then using an activity factor to account for your exercise levels and demands of your daily life. There are a vast number of BMR calculators available, however, the best 2 are the Müller et al. equation and the Harris-Benedict equation. The Müller et al. equation[4] is slightly more accurate as it accounts for lean mass and body fat and is my recommended choice. However, if you do not know your body fat percentage, the Harris-Benedict equation[5] is a good alternative but may slightly over-predict your BMR.

Müller et al.

(13.587 x Lean Body Mass) + (9.613 x Fat Mass) + (198 x Sex) - (3.351 x Age) + 674 = BMR

Note: for sex, Men = 1 and Women = 0

Mr Couch Potato:
    (13.587 x** 61.38 kg**) + (9.613 x** 31.62 kg**) + (198 x** 1**) - (3.351 x** 41 years**) + 674
    = 1,873 kcal/day

Miss Gym-Bunny:
    (13.587 x** 43.45 kg**) + (9.613 x** 11.55 kg**) + (198 x** 0**) - (3.351 x** 24 years**) + 674
    = 1,295 kcal/day

Harris-Benedict

Men: 88.362 + (13.397 x bodyweight in kg) + (4.799 x height in cm) - (5.677 x age) = BMR
Women: 447.593 + (9.247 x bodyweight in kg) + (3.098 x height in cm) - (4.330 x age) = BMR

Mr Couch-Potato:
    ***88.362 + (13.397 x** 93 kg**) + (4.799 x** 178 cm**) - (5.677 x** 41 years**) =** 1,956 kcal/day*

Miss Gym-Bunny:
    ***447.593 + (9.247 x** 55 kg**) + (3.098 x** 162 cm**) - (4.330 x** 24 years**) =** 1,354 kcal/day*

Activity Factor

Now that you have your BMR it's time to account for the calories you burn off through physical activity. To achieve this, we must multiply your BMR by an activity factor based upon how much you are exercising and how physical your daily life is. For example, a sedentary person engaged in no regular exercise needs far fewer calories than someone working a hard manual labour job and training regularly.

Multiplication Factor	Activity Level	Description
1.2	Sedentary	You work a desk-based job and don't exercise.
1.375	Lightly Active	You work a desk-based job but exercise 1-2 times/week or you don't exercise but have a pretty active job where you are on your feet for most of the day.
1.55	Moderately Active	You work a desk-based job but exercise 3-5 times/week or you have an active job where you are on your feet for most of the day AND exercise 1-2 times/week.
1.725	Highly Active	You work an active job where you are on your feet most of the day and exercise 3-5 times/week or more.
1.9	Extra Active	You work a hard manual labour job and are engaged in vigorous exercise 5+ days per week.

Now let's apply these activity factors to Mr Couch-Potato and Miss Gym-Bunny.

Mr Couch-Potato: **1,906 kcal/day x** 1.2 (Sedentary) **= TDEE of** 2,248 kcal/day

Miss Gym-Bunny: **1,295 kcal/day x** 1.725 (Highly Active) **= TDEE of** 2,234 kcal/day

Remember, your TDEE is the number of calories you need to consume to maintain your weight and you will need to eat above or below this maintenance amount to make changes to your weight. While it is possible to gain muscle mass and lose body fat within a calorie deficit, it is impossible to gain fat while in a calorie deficit.

Calories In

As stated at the beginning of this chapter the 'calories in' side of our equation consists of the total amount of food and drink you consume each day including alcohol. This is not to say that there aren't other factors that can affect this side of the equation i.e. hormones like Leptin and Ghrelin, genetics like the FTO gene, an obesigenic food environment, socioeconomics, sleep, stress, etc., but rather all of these factors potentially affect metabolic adaptations or influence how much food you consume by either affecting hunger levels, increasing the palatability of foods, or affecting your food choices, which leads to the overconsumption of calories. Put simply, carbs don't make you fat, fats don't make you fat, your hormones don't make you fat, eating too many calories (i.e. more than your TDEE) and not increasing your energy expenditure does make you fat.

Now that you understand all of the components of your TDEE and how to calculate your energy expenditure, it's time to learn about how your body uses energy to fuel exercise and the different energy pathways your body uses to produce energy for your working muscles.

Energy Continuum

Your muscles require energy to contract and generate movement. This energy comes in the form of *Adenosine Triphosphate (ATP)* and is the only form of energy that can be used by the muscles in the human body. ATP can be thought of as your body's energy currency in which all aspects of your life cost you energy and you must earn more (i.e. eat food) to meet your expenses (i.e. your TDEE). ATP consists of an

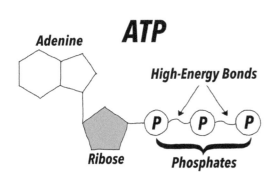

adenine base, with an attached sugar (ribose), and three phosphate molecules. The bonds between each of the phosphate molecules contain lots of energy which is released when each phosphate molecule is removed. When one phosphate is removed from ATP you are left with *Adenosine Diphosphate (ADP)* and when two phosphates are removed you are left with *Adenosine Monophosphate (AMP)*. This process can be reversed as long as there is sufficient energy available to replace the bonds. This required energy comes from your diet and each macronutrient has a different process to replenish ATP levels dependant on the duration and intensity of physical activity. The three sources for the replenishment of ATP are the *Phosphagen System*, *Glycolytic System*, and *Oxidative System*[6].

The Phosphagen System

The Phosphagen System utilises ATP and *Phosphocreatine (PCr)* stored in your muscle fibres. Phosphocreatine is found as creatine in meat and fish but is more effective when taken in supplement form as Creatine Monohydrate. With the help of the enzyme *Creatine Kinase*, PCr donates it's phosphates to ADP so it can be synthesised into ATP. This is the fastest of the energy systems and energy from this system is available for immediate use. However, the phosphagen system's ability to supply energy is limited and can only support all-out efforts of less than 30 seconds.

The Glycolytic System

The Glycolytic System (a.k.a The Anaerobic System) uses glucose or glycogen to produce ATP without the need for oxygen (**Anaerobic** = without oxygen). Without oxygen, lactate accumulates and can lead to muscle fatigue and as a result, the anaerobic system is used primarily for exercise lasting between 30 seconds and 3 minutes. The glycolytic system uses glycolysis to produce ATP (**Glyco** = glucose/glycogen **lysis** = breakdown). *Fast Glycolysis* is when *Pyruvate* (the end product of glycolysis) is converted into lactate, which is used to quickly produce ATP. Alternatively, lactate can enter the *Citric Acid Cycle* (or aerobic system) where it takes much longer to produce ATP and as a result is called *Slow Glycolysis*. The trade-off here is while fast glycolysis quickly produces ATP, it cannot produce as much ATP as slow glycolysis.

The Oxidative System

The oxidative system (a.k.a. The Aerobic System, **Aerobic** = with oxygen) can use carbs or fats to create ATP and in extreme situations, protein can be used too. Unlike the anaerobic system, the byproducts of the aerobic system do not cause fatigue. However, if inadequate amounts of oxygen are delivered to the muscles then your body will switch back to using the glycolytic system and blood lactate will accumulate. So long as there is sufficient levels of oxygen and enough macronutrients, the oxidative system can supply ATP to the working muscles for exercise bouts lasting from 3 minutes to many hours in length. The oxidative system occurs in the *Mitochondria* and has several different names including the Citric Acid Cycle, *Krebs Cycle* or the *Tricarboxylic Acid (TCA) Cycle*.

These three systems (a.k.a pathways) form an *Energy Continuum*, where each pathway overlaps with each other to ensure a constant ability to produce ATP to fuel muscular contractions. Each pathway produces ATP at decreasingly slower speeds and once one pathway's fuel source is depleted, the next pathway takes over and the intensity of exercise that can be maintained is naturally reduced. For example, once a long-distance marathon runner has depleted all their blood glucose and glycogen stores, their oxidative system will

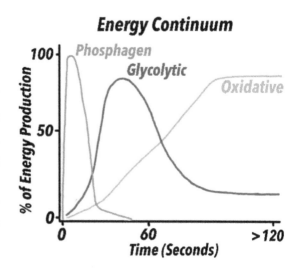

continue using fat but will produce half the amount of ATP, causing the runner to slow down due to decreased energy supplies. The limitations of these energy pathways are the reason why you cannot sprint a marathon at flat-out speed or lift heavy weights non-stop without rest.

Metabolism

So far we have discussed how many calories you "burn off" each day and how the body generates energy from your food, but we still need to address what exactly calories are and why they shouldn't be the only thing you focus on in your diet. A calorie in physics is a unit of heat generation. In food, *1 kilocalorie (kcal) equals how much energy it takes to heat 1 kilogram of water by 1 degree Celsius.* To assess how many calories a specific food item contains, the food of interest is placed into a bomb calorimeter, submerged in water and electrodes inserted into the food. The food is then electrocuted which burns the food and heats the water. The amount the water is heated equals how many calories the food item has. This is far from a perfect system and the actual calorie content of food items may vary greatly. Therefore, you should keep in mind that the calories stated on food packaging are only an estimate and you should expect some fluctuations between estimated and actual calorie content. Another key consideration is that 1 calorie of carbohydrates is not processed the same way as 1 calorie of fat or protein due to the different effects each macronutrient has on your hormones. Overall, the macronutrient balance of your meals, relative ease of digestion, feeding time, relative time to exercise, thermic effect of food, stress, and

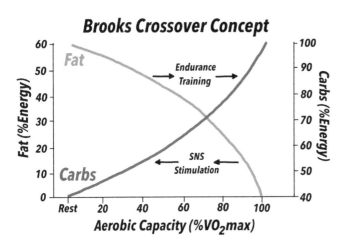

more can affect whether foods are stored as fat, converted to muscle tissue, or lost as heat. With performance, your metabolic efficiency is key to improving exercise tolerance and endurance. *Metabolic efficiency is your body's efficiency at utilising carbohydrate and fat stores at different intensities of exercise and rest*. A key concept on the topic of metabolic efficiency is the *Brooks Crossover Concept* which is the principle of where you will burn fat to a point then "switch" to burning more carbohydrates[7]. If you switch to burning more carbohydrates too early this may limit your ability to exercise at higher intensities/longer durations and increase your need to re-fuel during exercise to maintain your efforts. *Your metabolic efficiency can be improved through macronutrient periodisation where you maintain your protein intake and vary the relative proportion of your diet from fats and carbohydrates.* Improvements in metabolic efficiency can be achieved in as little as 7 days from dietary interventions but longer periods of 4 weeks are better for habit-forming. Around 75% of your metabolic efficiency is determined by your diet with the remaining 25% dictated by your exercise levels. For more information on macronutrient periodisation see the practical applications section of Chapter 2. Endurance training increases the length of time it takes to switch to preferentially burning carbohydrates and stimulation of the sympathetic nervous system (SNS) decreases the time to switch. Therefore, regular exercise, good recovery strategies, and taking care of your emotional well-being all improve your metabolic efficiency. The more efficient your metabolism becomes the lower your need for simple sugars to supplement energy demands, however, a highly efficient metabolism may lower your BMR and the number of calories burned during exercise. To summarise, we don't eat calories, we eat food. Therefore, you need to understand the basics of how each macronutrient is metabolised within your body so when we discuss macronutrient balance, meal frequency/timing, and bioavailability, you can make better diet and lifestyle choices to enhance your health and performance.

Carbohydrates

Dietary carbohydrates are broken down into glucose which moves freely in the bloodstream and then used to produce ATP through glycolysis. Glucose is also produced through the breakdown of stored glycogen through *Glycogenolysis*. Glucose is transported across the muscle membrane by a special transport protein called *GLUT4*, which is regulated by *Insulin*. Insulin is a hormone secreted by the β-islet cells of the pancreas. Without insulin, the cells are unaware of the glucose available in the blood and cannot utilise it for energy production. Insufficient levels of insulin or a resistance to its effects is a key step in the development of type 2 diabetes. If glucose remains unused in the bloodstream it will be stored as glycogen in the liver and muscles or will undergo lipogenesis (**lipo** = lipid/fat, **genesis** = creation) and stored as body fat. How different carbohydrates are metabolised can have a significant effect on energy production and your health in general. As insulin is an inhibitor to lipolysis (i.e. the breakdown of fat) consuming carbohydrates that limit the insulin response may help in weight management and diabetes risk. Carbohydrates that cause a low-insulin response are called *Low Glycaemic Index (Low-GI)* carbohydrates and those that have a high-insulin response are called *High Glycaemic Index (High-GI)* carbohydrates[8].

The glycaemic index of each food is compared to a reference food (typically white bread) and given a score where Low-GI carbohydrates score <55 and High-GI carbohydrates score >70. By consuming the majority of your carbohydrates from Low-GI carbohydrates you may limit the negative effects of excess insulin levels. As foods are not eaten in isolation mixing high and low-GI foods may help to lower your glucose response and prevent the potential negative effects of eaten high-GI foods. High-GI carbohydrates can still be used when a quicker source of energy is needed, like mid-exercise snacking during endurance events.

Example Low/High Glycaemic Index (GI) foods

Low-Glycemic Index Foods	High-Glycemic Index Foods
Broccoli (15)	White Bread (100)
Spaghetti (42)	Muesli (80)
Chickpeas (47)	Baked Potatoes (85)
Apples (38)	Watermelon (72)
Lentils (41)	Bagels (103)
Banana (54)	Taco Shells (97)

Low-GI foods <55, Moderate-GI foods 55-70, High-GI foods >70

Fat

Dietary fat is broken down by *Lipolysis* into glycerol and fatty acids. Fatty acids cannot travel within the bloodstream unassisted as they are hydrophobic (*hydro* = water, *phobic* = fear or aversion to something). Therefore, for fats to be used by the cells, the 3 (*tri*) fatty acids are first combined with glycerol during digestion or within the liver. This generates a helpful energy molecule called a *Triglyceride* (Trigs). Lipolysis is also regulated by insulin along with *Catecholamines* (specialist compounds that enable nerve signal transmission). The triglycerides are packaged into specialist fat globules called *Lipoproteins*, which form a kind of ship for the triglycerides, fat-soluble vitamins, and cholesterol to travel inside. The largest type of lipoproteins are the *Chylomicrons* which are created following meals. The second-largest are the *Very Low-Density Lipoproteins (VLDL)* which originate from the liver. Two other forms of lipoprotein you may have heard of are *Low-Density Lipoproteins (LDL)* and *High-Density Lipoproteins (HDL)*, which are the so-called "bad" and "good" cholesterol tested by your doctor during routine blood tests. Too much "bad" cholesterol and not enough "good" cholesterol may increase your risk of cardiovascular disease. The mobilisation of fatty acids within your body is regulated by *Lipoprotein Lipase* which is released by the endothelial cells in the region of the target adipose tissue (i.e. fat) or muscles. This triggers the lipoproteins to travel to the target site and release the fatty acids to be either stored in the adipocytes (i.e fat cells) several hours after eating or used by the muscle cells for energy production during exercise. The uptake of fatty acids by the muscle cells is regulated by the fatty acid transporters *Fatty Acid Binding Protein (FABP)*, *Fatty Acid Transport Protein (FATP)*, and *Fatty Acid Translocase (FAT or CD36)*. The greater the amount of these fatty acid transports the greater the uptake of fatty acids by your muscle cells and therefore the better your endurance fitness levels. Excess amounts of fatty acids can be converted into ketones, which are used to produce ATP through the citric acid cycle. Ketones are often increased in your body following prolonged exercise, reduced dietary carbohydrate intake, or fasting/starvation.

Protein

"Everything we do, everything we are, and everything we become depend on the action of thousands of different proteins". This quote by Michael Houston accurately sums up just how important protein is to our lives. Because protein is essential to life it is not considered a primary source of energy but can be utilised during periods of fasting, starvation, or caloric restriction. One gram of protein provides 4 kcal of energy and the average adult has around 10 - 12 kg of protein within the body, primarily as skeletal muscle tissue. Therefore, when utilising protein as an energy source you are basically eating your muscles, so you want to avoid that and eat enough protein. With protein metabolism, the most important factor to understand is the dynamic nature of *Protein Turnover*. The proteins within your body are in a constant state of flux where new proteins are being made through *Protein Synthesis* and old ones are being broken down in the gut into *Amino Acids* through *Protein Degradation.* Amino acids are absorbed and transported in the blood where they are deposited primarily in skeletal muscles and the liver. The liver is responsible for the production of non-essential amino acids (covered in Chapter 2) and is, therefore, key to regulating the delivery of amino acids into other tissues, not just muscle. The amino acids that are in the blood and the extracellular fluids are known as the *Free Amino Acid Pool.* As your body has no storage capabilities for protein the free amino acid pool is relatively small and is in a constant state of flux due to protein turnover. Excess proteins that are not utilised during protein synthesis are used to produce compounds that can enter the Citric Acid Cycle to produce energy. One key aspect of the breakdown of amino acids, is the production of urea during deamination. Deamination is the removal of the nitrogen-based compound ammonia from an amino acid to produce an α-keto acid for use in the oxidative systems. The urea produced during this process is excreted in the urine, with urea levels reaching 2 - 3 times the norm in athletes on a high-protein diet. Despite this increase in urea, high-protein diets pose no risk to your health with suggested buffers in dairy and alkaline vegetables serving to protect your body from any potential harm.

Practical Applications

When it comes to energy balance and metabolism the focus at this stage should fall solely on whether your goal is to lose body fat, gain muscle mass, or maintain your current body composition. To maintain your weight, you just need to calculate your TDEE and consume that amount of calories each day so this does not require any further explanation. We will also not look at trying to just lose or gain total weight as this is not practical for performance or general health.

Fat Loss

There are four core principles to effective/sustainable fat loss:

- Eat within a calorie deficit (Calories In is less than your TDEE)
- Follow a rate of weight loss between 0.5 - 1.0% of total bodyweight/week.
- Consume a high protein diet (i.e. 1.6 - 2.2 g/kg/day).
- Engage in 2+ resistance training sessions per week.

By following all four core principles you can optimise the amount of weight lost from body fat and minimise the amount lost from lean muscle mass. For example, while it is possible to lose weight at faster rates than 1% of total bodyweight per week (particularly in obese individuals), the percentage of weight loss from body fat will decrease with faster rates of weight loss and more muscle loss will occur. The same rules also apply to inactive individuals, those engaged in predominantly cardiovascular exercise, and individuals consuming low amounts of protein (i.e. < 1.6 g/kg/day) (see table below). To help you calculate your numbers, follow the 9-step method opposite toward efficient fat loss.

Approximate Ratio of Fat Mass loss to Lean Body Mass loss based on weight, diet, and exercise habits

	Normal Protein + No Resistance Training	High Protein + No Resistance Training	Normal Protein + Resistance Training	High Protein + Resistance Training
Obese	80/20	90/10	90/10	>90/<10
Overweight	70/30	80/20	80/20	90/10
Average	60/40	70/30	70/30	80/20
Lean	<50/>50	60/40	60/40	70/30

Table adapted from *Fat Loss Forever by Peter Baker & Layne Norton*[9]

Step 1.
Calculate your BMR using either the Müller et al. or Harris-Benedict equation.

Step 2.
Multiply your BMR by the most relevant activity factor to get your TDEE.

Step 3.
Decide on a rate of weekly weight loss between 0.5 and 1.0% of your total bodyweight.

Step 4.
Determine your approximate fat and muscle loss percentages using the table opposite.

Step 5.
Multiply your weekly weight loss in kg by each percentage for fat and muscle then multiply the total by 1,000 to convert to grams.

Step 6.
Multiply your fat loss in grams by 9 and multiple your muscle loss in grams by 4.

Step 7.
Add your protein and fat totals together to get your weekly calorie deficit.

Step 8.
Divide your weekly calorie deficit by 7 to get your daily calorie deficit.

Step 9.
Subtract your daily calorie deficit from your TDEE to get your daily target caloric intake.

To help explain we'll use our earlier Mr Couch-Potato example. Mr Couch-Potato wants to lose some excess body fat but isn't willing to exercise and doesn't want to follow a high protein diet (i.e. your typical yo-yo dieter). We have already calculated Mr Couch-Potato's TDEE but now we need to decide on a rate of weight loss taking into consideration a minimum number of calories he should consume to main good health (usually around 1,600 calories/day). Mr Couch-Potato isn't a fan of dieting and as such opts for a modest rate of weight loss of 0.5% of total bodyweight per week. The following calculations detail his requirements to meet his target.

- Mr Couch-Potato's TDEE = *2,284 calories/day*
- At 93 kg, a 0.5% per week rate of weight loss is approx. 0.5 kg or *500 g per week*.
- As Mr. Couch-Potato is obese, he can expect to lose around 80% of this weight from body fat and 20% from muscle mass.
- Therefore, 500 g per week will be 400 g from fat + 100 g from protein (muscle mass).
- There are 9 calories/gram of fat and 4 calories/gram of protein. Therefore, the total amount of calories needed to achieve the target 500 g = (400 g of fat x 9) + (100 g of protein x 4) = approx. 3,900 calories.
- We then divide this number by 7 to get his *daily calorie deficit of 557 calories*.
- So, in order to lose 0.5% of his total bodyweight per week, Mr. Couch-Potato should consume 557 fewer calories per day for a daily total of 1,727 calories (i.e. his TDEE of 2,284 calories – his daily deficit of 557 calories).

As Mr Couch-Potato's weight decreases the amount of weight which is equal to 0.5% of his weight will also decrease and these numbers will need to be recalculated. This is best done every 4 weeks for practicality. As Mr Couch-Potato gets closer and closer toward a healthy weight, the percentage of body fat he can lose without exercising or consume high protein levels will decrease as shown in the above table. Without starting an exercise plan Mr Couch-Potato is unlikely to maintain a healthy weight as prolonged dieting without concurrent resistance-based exercise causes metabolic adaptations that lower BMR and makes weight maintenance more difficult to achieve.[10,11]

Gaining Muscle Mass

Several factors affect how much lean muscle mass you can add including your training age, genetics, exercise stimulus, recovery, supplementation, and caloric intake. For now, we will focus on the areas that affect your caloric intake as the rest will be covered in detail in the Hypertrophy chapter of Volume 2 of this book series. The largest factor affecting hypertrophy (*hyper* = over, *trophy* = growth) and the number of calories you need to consume is your training age. Your training age is determined by how long you have been consistently lifting weights for and how much muscle mass you have already accrued. For example, in your first year of training, it is possible to gain up to 0.75 - 1kg of muscle per month (9 - 12kg/year). This rapid rate of potential muscle gain is often called "newbie gains" but it not sustainable as you get closer each year to your genetic muscular potential. Each year your potential gains decrease until you can potentially only gain up to 0.9 - 1.36 kg of muscle per year! While this may seem small, even 2 - 3 kg of muscle can drastically change your body shape[12].

1st Year	Potential gain of 9 – 12 kg (20 - 30lbs) of muscle mass (0.75 – 1 kg (2 - 3lbs)/month).
2nd Year	Potential gain of 4.5 – 5.5 kg (10 - 15lbs) of muscle mass (0.375 – 0.46 kg (1 - 2lbs)/month).
3rd Year	Potential gain of 2.27 – 2.72 kg (5 - 6lbs) of muscle mass/year (0.19 – 0.23 kg (0.4 - 0.5lbs)/month.
4th Year	Potential gain of 0.9 – 1.36 kg (2 - 3lbs) of muscle mass/year (monthly amount not worth calculating).

Note: these numbers are for men only. Women can expect significantly lower amounts.

This slowing of muscle mass accumulation is as you approach your drug-free genetic potential. Drug-free is an important distinction to make here as with the help of anabolic hormones (i.e. steroids) it is possible to reach very unnatural amounts of muscle mass way above your genetic potential, but not without sacrificing your health in the process. Your drug-free muscular potential can be estimated using a Fat-Free Mass Index (FFMI) calculation as described below.

Male FFMI
$$\textbf{(Weight (kg) x (1 – body fat \%/100)/Height (m)}^2\textbf{) + (6.1 x (1.8 – Height (m))}$$

Female FFMI
$$\textbf{Weight (kg) x (1 – body fat \%/100)/Height (m)}^2$$

Without pharmaceuticals and assuming a healthy body fat percentage, a maximum FFMI for a man is 25 kg/m^2 and 22 kg/m^2 for a woman[13]. If you have great natural muscle building genetics, then you could reach around 1 kg/m^2 above these ranges, however, anything higher than this is a strong indication of anabolic drug use or high body fat levels. To help explain this calculation we'll use our new friend Mr Hard-Gainer.

Fat-Free Mass Index (FFMI) Values and Typical Muscular Development

	Men	Women
Skinny / Low Musculature	Under 18.5	Under 14.0
Average	18.5 - 19.9	14.0 - 15.9
Athletic Individuals / Gym Users	20.0 - 21.9	16.0 - 17.9
Advanced Gym User / Distinctly Muscular	22.0 - 25.0	18.0 - 22.0
Indicative of Steroid Use	Over 25.0	Over 22.0

Note: These are less accurate if you have a body fat percentage of >15% (men) or > 25% women

Mr Hard-Gainer

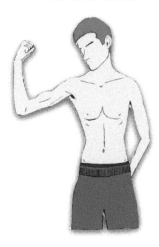

Age: **32**
Height: **175 cm**
Weight: **60 kg**
Body Fat: **9%**
Activity: **Sedentary job, just started resistance training 3/w**

Mr Hard-Gainer works in a sedentary job and has just started resistance training. He is currently very light for his height, with low amounts of muscle mass and low amounts of body fat. He is training consistently 3 times per week at the gym and wants to gain as much muscle mass as he can without getting fat.

Mr Hard-Gainer's FFMI = $((60 \text{ kg} \times (1 - 9\% / 100)) / (1.75\text{m} \times 1.75 \text{ m})) + (6.1 \times (1.8 - 1.75 \text{ m}))$

$= 18.14 \text{ kg/m}^2$

- Mr Hard-Gainer's TDEE = **2,416 calories/day**
- With a FFMI of 18.14 kg/m², and being a newcomer to resistance training, Mr Hard-Gainer has the potential to gain up to 9 -12 kg of lean muscle mass in his 1st year.
- 12 kg = 12,000 g. **12,000 g of muscle mass would take 48,000 calories to build** (12,000 x 4 cal/g protein). 48,000 calories divided by 365 days (1 year) = **approx. 132 cal/day**.
- Therefore, to optimise his energy balance for maximum muscle mass accumulation, Mr Hard-Gainer only needs 132 calories per day above his TDEE. However, it is recommended to **add 250 - 500 calories per day** to allow for fluctuations/errors in calculations (i.e. TDEE of 2,416 cal/d + 500 cal/d = 3,116 cal/d).
- Gym newbies or those with low FFMI scores should start with the higher end of this range and more experienced lifters the lower end. If Mr Hard-Gainer starts gaining fat very quickly then he should lower his surplus by 100 cal/d and continue to monitor.

You can gain muscle mass while in a calorie deficit as long as you are meeting your protein requirements, but, you cannot optimise muscle protein synthesis while in a calorie deficit. However, while it is possible to gain muscle mass while losing weight, as long as you're consuming enough protein, the amount of muscle mass you gain will not be as much when compared to eating a moderate calorie surplus. Notice I said moderate surplus. Traditional "bulking" diets recommend eating as much as you can every day, with the idea that more food equals more muscle. But, as you now know, how much muscle mass you can gain and how quickly you can gain it is limited, so eating more calories than needed to support this amount of muscle mass accumulation will just lead to excess fat mass as explained with our Mr Hard-Gainer example.

Where Should I Start?

At different stages of your life and athletic career, you may want to lose weight or gain weight to enhance your performance. However, if your focus is currently on improving your health then you may feel stuck on where to start. Should you try to gain as much muscle as you can before trying to cut down excess body fat (i.e. the typical bulking and cutting cycle), or should you be focusing on losing that spare tyre around your waist first? My recommendations here are to first check your Body Mass Index (BMI), waist circumference, and body fat percentage. If your BMI, waist circumference, and/or body fat are in the overweight/obese range (see tables below) then start with losing fat. If you are in the healthy range or underweight, focus on gaining muscle mass.

BMI (kg/m^2)			
Ethnicity	Healthy	Underweight/Overweight	Obese
Non-Asian Populations	18.5 – 24.9	<18.5 or 25.0 – 29.9	30.0+
Asian Populations	18.5 – 22.9	<18.5 or 23.0 – 27.4	27.5+

Note: Asian populations includes all South and East Asian ethnic groups. It does not include Northern Asian (i.e. Russian, -stan countries, or Middle Eastern countries)

Waist Circumference (cm)			
Ethnicity	Healthy	Overweight	Obese
Non-Asian Men	<94	94 – 102	>102
Asian Men	<90		>90
Non-Asian Women	<80	80 – 88	>88
Asian Women	<80		>80

Note: Best practice is to measure the waist at the narrowest part between the top of the hip bone and bottom rib, approx. 2-3 cm above the belly-button. There are no overweight "amber" ranges for Asian men and women due to the association between increases in waist circumference and a drastic increase in disease risk with values above 90 cm and 80 cm respectively.

Body Fat Percentage (%)			
Men (Age)	Healthy	Overweight	Obese
20 - 39	7.0 - 19.9	20.0 - 24.9	>25.0
40 - 59	10.0 - 21.9	22.0 - 28.4	>28.5
60 - 79	12.0 - 24.9	25.0 - 29.9	>30.0
Women (Age)			
20 - 39	21.0 - 32.9	33.0 - 39.4	>39.5
40 - 59	23.0 - 33.9	34.0 - 39.9	>40.0
60 - 79	24.0 - 34.9	35.0 - 41.4	>41.5

Note: Body fat values under the healthy range may occur in very lean physique athletes however, essential body fat for men is 3% and for women is 13%. Levels below this are dangerously low and may cause health complications. Additionally, FFMI calculations are only accurate with healthy bodyweight. Therefore, if your body fat is within the overweight or obese range consider focusing more on losing excess fat before considering your maximum muscular potential.

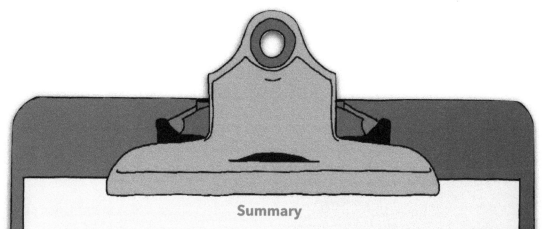

Summary

✓ Energy balance is the balance between how many calories you consume and the amount you expend a.k.a. **Calories In vs Calories Out**.

✓ Weight loss is the product of a negative calorie balance (i.e. Calories In < Calories Out), whereas weight gain is the product of a positive calorie balance (i.e. Calories In > Calories Out).

✓ The estimated number of calories you expend or per day is called your **Total Daily Energy Expenditure (TDEE)** and is comprised of your **Basal Metabolic Rate (BMR)**, **Non-Exercise Activity Thermogenesis (NEAT)**, **The Thermic Effect of Food**, and **Exercise Activity**.

✓ Your BMR can be estimated using mathematical calculations such as the Müller et al. or Harris-Benedict calculations. These can then be multiplied by an activity factor to calculate your TDEE.

✓ Your cells need energy to perform their work which comes from **Adenosine Triphosphate (ATP)**.

✓ There are 3 sources for replenishing ATP: the **Phosphagen System**, **Glycolytic System**, and **Oxidative System**.

✓ The Phosphagen System replenishes ATP quickly but can only support activities less than 30 seconds in length. The Glycolytic System replenishes energy slower but can support activities up to 3 minutes in length. The Oxidative system is the slowest but can continue to produce ATP for hours, as long as there is enough food supplies to support it.

✓ All 3 energy systems work together to form an **Energy Continuum** which ensures ATP can always be replenished. However, the longer the activity, the lower the intensity that can be maintained due to the slower nature of ATP production and the accumulation of Lactate.

✓ Your body utilises carbohydrates and fats as fuel. The intensity and duration of the activity determines how much of each nutrient is used. The more endurance exercise you engage in, the better your body becomes at utilising fat to fuel activity before needing to deplete carbohydrate stores. Whereas, poor recovery, stress, and stimulants may decrease the time it takes to switch to preferentially burning carbohydrates.

✓ Carbohydrates are broken down through digestion into sugars. With the help of the hormone **Insulin**, these sugars (a.k.a. Glucose) is taken up by the cells and used to generate ATP. Fats are broken down through digestion and packaged with sugars into energy molecules called **Triglycerides**, which contain both fats and sugar and travel in special "ships" called lipoproteins. Protein is used as the building blocks for all life. Dietary protein is broken down into Amino Acids to form the **Free Amino Acid Pool**, which is in constant flux due to protein breakdown and protein synthesis.

✓ The maximum amount of muscle mass you can add to your body without using anabolic hormones or other dangerous substances can be calculated using a **Fat-Free Mass Index (FFMI)** calculator. The maximum FFMI for a drug-free man and women is 25 kg/m² and 22 kg/m² respectively.

REFERENCES

[1] Trexler, E.T., Smith-Ryan, A.E. & Norton, L.E. (2014), *Metabolic adaptation to weight loss: implications for the athlete*. Journal of the International Society of Sports Nutrition 11, 7. https://doi.org/10.1186/1550-2783-11-7

[2] Calcagno, M., Kahleova, H., Alwarith, J., Burgess, N. N., Flores, R. A., Busta, M. L., & Barnard, N. D., (2019), *The Thermic Effect of Food: A Review*, Journal of the American College of Nutrition, 38:6, 547-551, https://doi.org/10.1080/07315724.2018.1552544

[3] Ainsworth, B. E., Haskell, W. L., Herrmann, S. D., Meckes, N., Bassett, D. R. JR., Tudor-Locke, C., Greer. J. L., Vezina, E. J., Whitt-Glover, M. C., Leon, A. (2011), *2011 Compendium of Physical Activities: A Second Update of Codes and MET Values*, Medicine & Science in Sports &Exercise, 43(8) 1575 - 1581, https://doi.org/10.1249/MSS.0b013e31821ece12

[4] Müller B, Merk S, Bürgi U, Diem P., (2001) *Calculating the basal metabolic rate and severe and morbid obesity*, Praxis (Bern 1994). 8;90(45):1955-63

[5] Roza, A. M., and Shizgal, H. M., (1984), *The Harris Benedict equation reevaluated: resting energy requirements and the body cell mass*, The American Journal of Clinical Nutrition, 40(1), 168–182, https://doi.org/10.1093/ajcn/40.1.168

[6] MacLaren, D. and Morton, J. (2012), *Biochemistry for Sport and Exercise Metabolism*, Wiley-Blackwell

[7] Antonio, J. et al. (2008), *Essentials of Sports Nutrition and Supplements*, Humana Press

[8] Opperman, A. M., Venter, C. S., Oosthuizen, W., Thompson, R. L., and Vorster, H. H., (2004), *Meta-analysis of the health effects of using the glycaemic index in meal-planning*, 92(3), 367-381, https://doi.org/10.1079/BJN20041203

[9] Baker, P. and Norton, L. E. (2019), *Fat Loss Forever*, Independently Published

[10] Dulloo A. G., Jacquet J., Montani J. P., (2012), *How dieting makes some fatter: from a perspective of human body composition autoregulation*, Proceedings of the Nutrition Society. 71(3): 379-89. https://doi.org/10.1017/S0029665112000225

[11] Maclean, P.S., Bergouignan, A., Cornier, M. A.,and Jackman, M., (2011),: *Biology's response to dieting: the impetus for weight regain*. American Journal of Physiology Regulatory, Integrative and Comparative Physiology. 301: R581-R600. https://doi.org/10.1152/ajpregu.00755.2010

[12] Schoenfeld, B., (2016), *Science and Development of Muscle Hypertrophy*, Human Kinetics, New York

[13] Kouri, E. M., Pope, H. G. Jr., Katz, D. L., and Oliva, P., (1995), *Fat-free mass index in users and nonusers of anabolic-androgenic steroids*, Clinical Journal of Sport Medicine: 5(4): 223-228, https://doi.org/10.1097/00042752-199510000-00003

2

MACRONUTRIENTS

What are they and why do you need them?

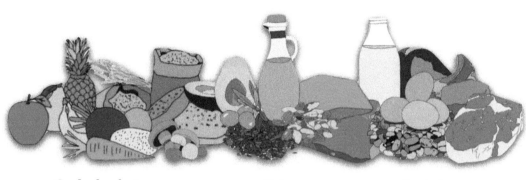

Carbohydrates   **Fats**   **Protein**

Macronutrients (***macro*** = large) are types of food that are required by the body in large quantities. The three different macronutrients are *Carbohydrates*, *Fat*, and *Protein*. A nutrition plan with tailored macronutrient content can help to decrease your risk of illness and injury, as well as maximise your training adaptations and improve your performance.

Carbohydrates

Carbohydrates (a.k.a. **Carbs** or **Saccharides**) are your body's primary source of fuel during moderate to vigorous exercise. Carbohydrates are sometimes abbreviated as CHO, which represents their molecular structure of Carbon, Hydrogen, and Oxygen[1]. Carbohydrates are not an essential macronutrient as they can be created through the breakdown of other non-carbohydrate sources, through a process called *gluconeogenesis* (***gluco*** = sugar, ***genesis*** = creation). Carbohydrates provide 4 kcal/gram of energy and improve performance by increasing *glycogen* stores in the liver and muscles, increasing work capacity (i.e. how long you can exercise for). However, your body has limited stores for glycogen and excess dietary calories from carbohydrates will be stored as body fat. Carbohydrate intake can vary greatly with typical intakes ranging from very low (<50g/day) to high (>400g/day)[2]. Low-carb diets may aid in achieving weight loss goals or improve metabolic efficiency[3] but conversely, very low-carb diets (a.k.a. Keto diets) may cause health complications for diabetic patients due to prolonged ketosis[4] (the production of ketones as a substitute energy source for your brain). For the potential benefits and limitations of restricting or increasing carbohydrate intake, see the practical applications section. Carbohydrates come in four different forms: *Monosaccharides*, *Disaccharides*, *Oligosaccharides*, and *Polysaccharides*.

Monosaccharides

Monosaccharides (*mono* = 1, *saccharide* = sugar) include *ribose* and *deoxyribose*, which form an essential part of your DNA, as well as *glucose*, *fructose*, and *galactose*, which are *"simple sugars"* obtained from your diet.

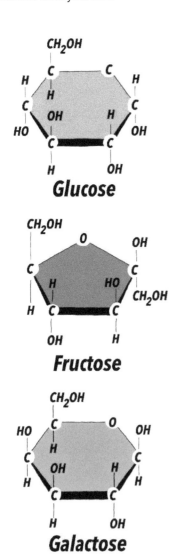

Glucose

Fructose

Galactose

Glucose is the end product of when larger carbohydrates are broken down during digestion and serve as the primary source of energy in the body. Glucose circulates in the bloodstream where it is transported to the muscles, brain, or internal organs. If not immediately needed, glucose can also be stored as *Glycogen* in the muscles and to a lesser extent the liver. Found naturally in a variety of food sources, glucose is sometimes referred to as Dextrose and simply blood sugar when in the bloodstream. How well regulated the sugar (i.e. glucose) is in your blood is a key factor in your risk of developing type 2 diabetes[5].

Fructose (a.k.a. Levulose or "Fruit Sugar") is a monomer of glucose (i.e. they both have the same chemical formula $C_6H_{12}O_6$). However, fructose cannot be used in its natural form and must be converted into glucose within the liver[6]. Fructose is found naturally in small quantities in fruit and vegetables but is added to several processed foods in much higher quantities, often in the form of high-fructose corn syrup (HFCS). When eaten as part of whole fruit or small quantities of honey, fructose is not harmful to your health[7]. However, when eaten in high volume as part of more heavily processed foods, which do not include the fibre and other key nutrients that affect how fructose behaves in your body, fructose can be detrimental to health and may increase your risk of non-alcoholic fatty liver disease and diabetes[8].

Galactose is another monomer of glucose and is combined with glucose to make the disaccharide lactose. Much like fructose, galactose cannot be used in its natural form and first needs to be converted into glucose within the liver.

Disaccharides

Disaccharides (**di** = 2) including **sucrose**, **lactose**, and **maltose**, are composed of 2 simple sugars joined together.

Sucrose is a combination of glucose and fructose and its crystallised form is found in large quantities in sugar beets, sugar cane, and maple syrup. There are many common names for sucrose including table sugar, beet sugar, or cane sugar. Sucrose is also found in most fruit and vegetables in varying amounts. Sucrose is often purified and packaged as white, brown, and powdered sugars. However, despite these different purified varieties, excess calories from sugar consumption, regardless of its type, can have a detrimental effect on your health. Sucrose is used in the production of some artificial sweeteners, which are potentially healthy alternatives to sugar as they contain low/no calories. Artificial sweeteners have previously raised concerns over potential increased cancer and diabetes risk. However, more recent reviews of the research have shown no significant correlation between artificial sweeteners and cancer or diabetes.[9, 10]

Lactose is a combination of galactose and glucose and is found only in the milk of mammals (e.g. breast milk, cows milk, goats milk, etc.). Lactose intolerance is a genetic inability to properly digest lactose that can result in uncomfortable digestive symptoms. Infants are well adapted to digest lactose, as newborns receive all of their required nutrients through their mother's breast milk and have abundant amounts of the digestive enzyme *lactase*. As we

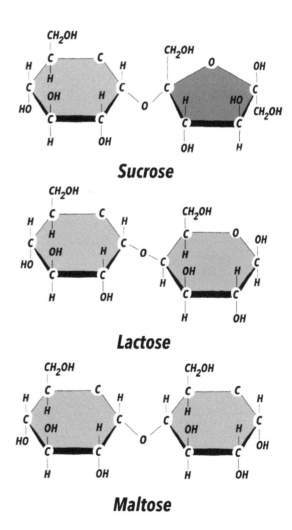

Sucrose

Lactose

Maltose

develop into adulthood this ability to digest lactose is sometimes lost due to declining levels of the lactase enzyme. However, approximately 8,000-10,000 years ago in the region of modern-day Turkey the first adults able to digest lactose were recorded, due to a favourable mutation of the MCM6 gene[11]. This mutation spread across Europe and beyond with up to 98% of Europeans possessing this favourable gene mutation and can digest lactose well. However, some areas of Asia have a 100% incidence of lactose intolerance due to a lack of the MCM6 gene. While lactose intolerance is primarily genetic, poor biodiversity of the *Gut Microbiome* or injury to the intestines may also cause lactose intolerance[12]. Improving your diet diversity may eliminate food intolerances by improving your gut microbiome, discussed in detail in Chapter 6.

Maltose comprises of 2 glucose molecules bonded together and is formed when larger polysaccharides are broken down during digestion. Produced in nature, maltose occurs when seeds sprout and is important in initiating plant growth. This sprouting process is altered through heat in a process called malting. Malting is the first step used in the production of some alcoholic beverages, most notably beer. Very few food and drinks contain maltose other than alcoholic beverages; however, sweet potatoes are a healthy source of maltose[13].

Simple sugars are not inherently bad and do serve a purpose in performance and health. The primary concern around simple sugars should be their overall quantity in your diet and origin. Wherever possible aim for natural, minimally processed, and unrefined sources of simple sugars to maximise their health and performance benefits and limit potential risks. You should also try to ensure the majority of your carbohydrates are from complex carbohydrates, which we'll cover next.

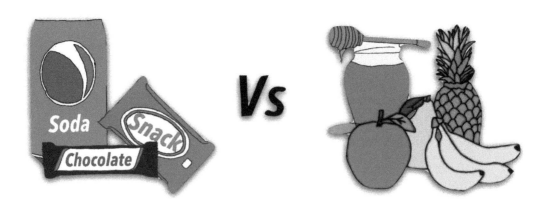

Oligosaccharides

Oligosaccharides (**oligo** = a few) are composed of 3-9 combined simple sugars and include **raffinose** and **inulin**. Along with Polysaccharides, these types of carbohydrates are known as "*complex carbohydrates*".

Raffinose is the family name of oligosaccharide compounds found primarily in beans, broccoli, wholegrains, cabbage, and asparagus. The most common of these compounds are *raffinose* (a trisaccharide) and *stachyose* (a tetrasaccharide), which both contain different combinations of the simple sugars glucose, galactose, and fructose. Raffi nose compounds have typically lower nutritional value due to poor digestibility. However, they serve as a benefi cial source of prebiotics for the gut microbiota[14].

Inulin (not to be confused with Insulin) is a form of stored energy, produced in plants and similar to that of glycogen in humans. Inulin is a type of fi bre, which aids in digestion and like raffi nose serves as a prebiotic for the gut microbiota[15]. Quality sources of inulin include chicory root, artichokes, asparagus, bananas, wholewheat grains, garlic, and leeks[16]. While inulin supplements are available, it is still much more effective when derived from a healthy diet.

Polysaccharides

Polysaccharides (**poly** = many) contain between 10 and thousands of glucose units and come from both plant and animal sources. The most important types of polysaccharides are *starch*, *fibre*, and *glycogen*.

Glycogen is the storage form of glucose and is stored in small quantities within the liver and skeletal muscles[17]. In total, there is approximately 15 g of glycogen stored within the body per kg of bodyweight. As a result of these relatively small stores, glycogen is only used as a temporary source of energy. Once depleted, your body will switch back to using fat stores as its primary source of energy. As the body's capacity to store glycogen is limited, excess glucose is converted into fat and stored around the body either viscerally (i.e. around the organs) or subcutaneously (i.e. under the skin). Glycogen metabolism plays a key role in the regulation of blood sugar levels working in partnership with the hormone insulin. Insulin promotes the storage of glucose as glycogen, as well as promoting glucose uptake by the cells and glycolysis. Maximising your glycogen stores is important to optimising your performance, regardless of whether you engage in high-intensity, short-duration sports or longer lower-intensity endurance sports[18].

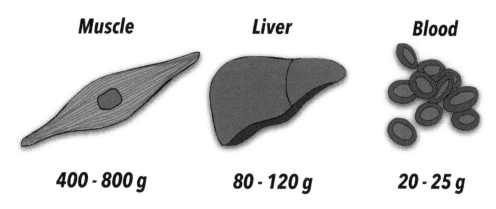

Muscle	Liver	Blood
400 - 800 g	**80 - 120 g**	**20 - 25 g**

For every 1 g of glycogen stored in the liver and muscles, an additional 3 g of water are stored. Therefore, 500 g of stored glycogen would equal a weight gain of 2 kg (500 g of glycogen + 1.5 kg of water). When in a calorie deficit or starting a low-carb diet you will often see a rapid rate of weight loss to begin with but slows after a week or so. This rapid weight loss is due to losing the water stored with your glycogen and not all fat loss. As discussed in Chapter 1, glycogen is utilised during longer bouts of exercise and in some energy pathways lead to the production of lactate. However, lactate can be converted into pyruvate and then back into glycogen once exercise intensity decreases or stops altogether.

Starch is the storage form of carbohydrates in plants and is found in 2 forms: *Amylose* and *Amylopectin*. Amylose makes up roughly 30% of the starch in all plants whereas amylopectin makes up the remaining 70%. The ratio between amylose and amylopectin within food sources helps determine its digestibility[19]. For example, foods with a relatively high proportion of amylopectin are digested well and increase the speed of absorption of other nutrients in the diet, whereas foods with relatively higher amylose are digested poorly which slows the absorption of other nutrients from the diet. This helpful regulation of the rate of absorption is important to ensure the nutrients in your diet have the right amount of time to be properly absorbed and utilised. Starch does not complete this job alone, in fact, it is more of a supporting player to dietary fibre.

Fibre is classified as a structural non-starch polysaccharide. Fibre is found in the cell walls of leaves, stems, roots, and seeds, and contains different types of fibre that act differently in your body, depending on whether or not they are soluble in water. As a result, fibre is often divided into 2 types: *Soluble Fibre* and *Insoluble Fibre*. Soluble fibres include *Psyllium*, *Pectin*, *Beta-Glucan*, and *Guar Gum* whereas insoluble fibres include: *Cellulose*, *Hemicellulose*, *Lignin*, and *Chitin*. Dietary fibre aids in digestion by providing bulk to the food residues that pass through the intensities[20]. It achieves this by holding onto large amounts of water. This is why good hydration is important for maintaining healthy digestion. Individually, the soluble fibre shortens the time food residues take to travel through the intensities (a.k.a. transit time), whereas the insoluble fibre helps the food residues to "scrape" along the lining of the intensities to aid in nutrient absorption. Fibre causes similar satiating effects as protein and is therefore helpful during weight loss efforts[21]. Good sources of soluble fibre include oats, whole grain rice, vegetables and fruits. Good sources of insoluble fibre include wholewheat bread and flour, vegetables, and wholegrains.

	Soluble Fibre		Insoluble Fibre
Psyllium	Also known as ispaghula and found in the husks of Plantago ovata plant seeds, psyllium is a bulk-forming laxative and a prebiotic with links to reduced heart disease and diabetes risk.	**Cellulose**	Cellulose gives plant cell walls their stiffness and strength. Cellulose is used in several manufacturing processes including textiles and paper production. Cellulose forms a large majority of bulk to your stools aiding digestion.
Pectin	Found in fruits and is often used in medicine to treat high cholesterol. Pectin is also used as a thickening agent in cooking and some denture adhesive.	**Hemicellulose**	Found in plant cell walls with similar functions as cellulose. Hemicellulose, however, consists of shorter chains of between 500 – 3,000 glucose units compared to cellulose's much longer 7,000 – 15,000 glucose units.
Beta-Glucan	Foods and supplements containing beta-glucans have been shown to lower heart disease risk, improve blood glucose regulation, and boosts your immune system. Beta-glucans are found in whole grains, oats, wheat, barley, fungi and some yeasts.	**Lignin**	Lignin (**lignum** = wood) is a large constituent of wood that may alter the rate of absorption and metabolism of nutrients in the diet. While not strictly considered a form of carbohydrates it is a good source of insoluble fibre found in root vegetables, flaxseed, wheat bran and more.
Guar Gum	Also known as guaran, guar gum is frequently used as a food additive to thicken and bind products. Guar gum in healthy doses can aid in digestive health by acting as a prebiotic, lowers blood sugar levels, reduces cholesterol, and aids weight loss through increasing satiety. High dose supplements of guar gum may be harmful to health and are best avoided.	**Chitin**	Forms the primary component of arthropod exoskeletons (i.e. crabs, lobsters, shrimps etc.), and performs a similar function to the protein keratin in mammals (needed to form hair and nails). Used to make products thicker and stiffer, chitin is used in both food and pharmaceutical products and some health food supplements as the compound chitosan. Chitin is primarily used for lowering cholesterol and improving kidney function.

Table References[22,23,24,25,26,27,28]

Fat

There are three types of lipids: *Simple Lipids*, which are Fats (including dietary fat) and Waxes; *Compound Lipids*, which include Phospholipids, Glycolipids, and Lipoproteins; and *Derived Lipids*, which includes steroids and other compounds[29]. Lipids are stored in adipose tissue (i.e. body fat), in the muscles as *Triglycerides* (a.k.a. *Triacylglycerols*), and in the blood as *Lipoproteins*. Triglycerides are too large to be used directly and need to be broken down through a process called **Lipolysis** into usable products called **Fatty Acids** and **Glycerol**. Fatty acids are hydrophobic (**hydro** = water, **phobic** = fear or aversion), and as a result, need some help to move around the body as humans are between 45% and 70% water. To achieve this, 3 fatty acids will attach to 1 glycerol molecule (a.k.a. a *glycerol backbone*), to form a very helpful energy molecule of both sugar and fat. Fat provides 9 kcal/gram of energy, more than double that of carbohydrates and protein. Much like carbohydrates, fat is composed of Carbon, Hydrogen, and Oxygen but are much larger with the "average" fat molecule having a chemical formula of $C_{55}H_{104}O_6$. There are many more different types of fat than carbohydrates due to variations in:

- **Saturation** (how many of the available chemical bonds are being used)
- **Double-bond positions** (parts of the fat where carbon binds with another carbon instead of hydrogen or oxygen)
- **Fatty acid placement** (where the fatty acids attach to the glycerol backbone)
- **Chain length** (how many fatty acids are in one fat molecule)

Based on saturation, dietary fats are divided into **Saturated Fats**, **Monounsaturated Fats**, and **Polyunsaturated Fats**. The fourth type of fat is primarily found in highly processed foods called **Trans-Modified Fats** and is classified by the abnormal position of its double bonds, causing the fatty acids to be more easily packed together. Unlike carbohydrates, some fats are needed in the diet as they cannot be produced within the body. These needed dietary fats are called **Essential Fatty Acids**.

Fat is the default fuel source in humans at rest and low-intensity exercise due to its relative abundance even in healthy weight individuals. Although each person has a "set point" of body fat that is tightly maintained over adult life[30], everyone still has a limitless ability to store body fat. Even in a lean athlete, body fat stores can hold approximately 30,000 – 40,000 calories of available fuel, enough to complete multiple marathons or weeks of resistance training sessions. Fat is not just an inert stored source of fuel, it also plays a significant role in your health and performance, with hormonal effects that include anti-inflammatory benefits, anti-depressive effects, anti-catabolic effects (*catabolic* = tissue breakdown), and more[31].

Saturated Fats

Saturated fats (**saturated** = containing as much as possible) are fat molecules where every single bond between its carbon atoms are being occupied, and the fat molecule is full (or saturated). Bonds are high energy links between elements caused by strong attractive forces, similar to how a magnet attracts metal objects. Carbon can form four bonds with other elements. For example, a carbon atom can bond with four hydrogen atoms to form the chemical Methane (CH_4). However, carbon can sometimes form more than one bond with other elements like when one carbon atom makes two double bonds with two oxygen atoms to form Carbon Dioxide (CO_2). Single bonds are stronger than double bonds making the molecule harder to breakdown. This is partly why saturated fats like butter and coconut oil are solid at room temperature. For many years, scientists have thought that saturated fats contribute to

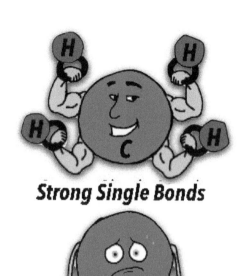

Strong Single Bonds

Weak Double Bonds

cardiovascular disease (CVD) risk by increasing the amount of Low-Density Lipoprotein (LDL) cholesterol in your body. However, current research shows that saturated fats alone do not increase CVD risk although this remains a widely researched and debated topic[37]. When the inner lining of your arteries become damaged through inflammation, LDL particles may penetrate the arterial wall and start to form fatty plaques which project into the artery, making the space for the blood to pass through smaller. This process is called *Atherosclerosis* and is the precursor to all cardiovascular diseases including heart attacks and strokes[32]. Not all saturated fats have the same level of impact on your CVD risk, with some saturated fats being less atherogenic (*atherogenic* = contributes to atherosclerosis), than others and may even be beneficial to your health and performance[33]. Saturated fat is found mostly in high-fat animal products such as fatty cuts of meat, "dark meat" poultry, and full-fat dairy. Plant sources of saturated fats include palm oil and coconut oil. Palm oil is commonly added to other foods to help them keep their shape, reduce costs, or make production easier. Being aware of the different names of individual fatty acids (see table overleaf) can help you to make better diet choices to fuel your performance and keep you in good health.

Palmitic Acid is the most common form of saturated fat in plants and animals and may comprise over 50% of the saturated fat in typical western diets[34]. Palm oil has the highest concentration of Palmitic Acid but it can also comprise up to a quarter of the saturated fats found in red meat and dairy. Palm oil is used as an additive in processed foods including some nut butters. Palmitic acid raises LDL cholesterol levels but the potential negative effects of this can be offset with increased omega-3 fatty acid intake (see polyunsaturated fats).

Stearic Acid is the second most common saturated fat in western diets but unlike some other saturated fats does not appear to negatively affect cholesterol levels[35]. Your body can convert stearic acid into Oleic acid but potentially not enough to have a significant effect on health. Stearic acid is mostly found in animal fat but also coconut oil and cocoa butter.

Myristic Acid has the most significant negative impact on LDL cholesterol levels out of all the saturated fats but is relatively rare and not found in high amounts in most foods[36].

Lauric Acid has a positive impact on your cholesterol profile by increasing High-Density Lipoprotein (HDL) cholesterol[37]. Lauric acid makes up approximately 42% of coconut oil and 47% of palm kernel oil.

Caproic, *Caprylic*, and *Capric Acid* derive their names from the Latin word "Capra" meaning goat because they are all abundant in goats milk.

Butyric, *Propionic*, and *Acetic Acid* are formed by your gut bacteria when they ferment fibre in your colon. The Starch, Pectin, and Inulin discussed earlier all promote the formation of these healthy saturated fatty acids.

Names of Common Saturated Fatty Acids		
Palmitic Acid	Stearic Acid	Myristic Acid
Lauric Acid	Capric Acid	Caprylic Acid
Caproic Acid	Butyric Acid	Propionic Acid
	Acetic Acid	

Monounsaturated Fats

Monounsaturated fats are fatty acids which contain one double bond in its chain. For example, *Oleic Acid* (a.k.a. *omega-9*) has one double bond between its 9th and 10th carbon atoms. Oleic Acid is found in very high amounts in olive oil. Regular consumption of olive oil has been linked to a significant decrease in CVD risk[38] and forms a central part of the Mediterranean Diet. Monounsaturated fats are generally seen as being healthier than saturated fats, however, some trans-modified versions of monounsaturated fats are more harmful to your health. One example is Trans-Elaidic Acid which is found in pastries like croissants and

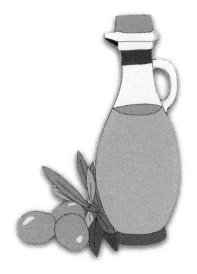

doughnuts. *Trans-Elaidic Acid* is also an omega-9 fatty acid but the double bonds occur on the opposite side to the normal (cis-) positioning. Therefore, the fatty acid does not curve with the double bonds and more fatty acids can be packed tightly together. Naturally occurring trans-modified fats such as those found in dairy and meat are not harmful to health. Artificial trans-fats, however, are harmful to your health by increasing inflammation and LDL cholesterol[39] and are added to processed foods to increase shelf life or keep foods solid at room temperature.

An example of a curved *cis*-**fat** like those found in healthy plant and animal fat sources.

Straight ***trans*-fat** with its abnormal double-bond, found predominantly in processed, man-made foods.

Names of Common Monounsaturated Fatty Acids		
Lauroleic Acid	Myristoleic Acid	Palmitoleic
Oleic Acid (omega-9)	Elaidic Acid	Vaccenic
Petroselinic Acid	Gadoleic Acid	Gondoic
Euricic Acid	Nervonic Acid	

Polyunsaturated Fats

Polyunsaturated fats are fatty acids with 2 or more carbon-carbon double bonds. Polyunsaturated fats include 2 essential fatty acids: *Linoleic Acid* (a.k.a. *omega-3*) and *Alpha-Linolenic Acid (ALA)* (a.k.a. *omega-6*). These fatty acids are considered essential as the body cannot produce sufficient amounts of them and they need to be obtained directly from the diet. Without sufficient amounts of omega-3 and omega-6 fatty acids, you can suffer from retarded growth, kidney issues, skin conditions, or even death[40]. Omega-3 fatty acids are found in fatty fish (salmon, mackerel, tuna, etc.), nuts, seeds, and avocados. Omega-6 fatty acids are found in soya beans, sunflower oil, corn oil, and are generally higher in processed foods. The balance between omega-3 and omega-6 fatty acids is also an important aspect as your body will preferentially absorb

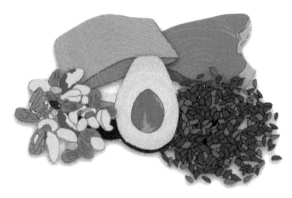

more omega-6 than omega-3. Therefore, it is recommended to consume a diet with a ratio of 7:1 (omega-6:omega-3) to ensure adequate levels are achieved[41]. The typical western diet consumes a much less favourable ration of closer to 20:1. Like oleic acid, the omega names of these essential fats come from the position of the carbon-carbon double bonds along its chain. For example, omega-3 has its first double bond between the 3rd and 4th carbon atoms and omega-6 between its 6th and 7th. Two additional omega-3 fatty acids are not strictly considered essential as they can be synthesised in the body from omega-6. These additional omega-3 fatty acids are called *Eicosapentaenoic Acid (EPA)* and *Docosahexaenoic Acid (DHA)*. EPA is needed for the development of several key growth hormones. DHA is needed for healthy brain and visual function and forms a major part of your brain's grey matter. Both EPA and DHA have been shown to reduce inflammation, improve blood pressure, decrease heart attack risk, improve mental health, and aid in recovery[42,43,44]. Fatty fish is the best source of both EPA and DHA.

Names of Common Polyunsaturated Fatty Acids		
Linoleic Acid (Omega-3)	Gamma-Linolenic-Acid	Dihomo-y-Linolenic Acid
Arachidonic Acid	Adrenic Acid	n-6 Docosapentaenoic Acid
Alpha-Linolenic-Acid (Omega-6)	Stearidonic Acid	Eicosapentaenoic Acid (EPA)
n-3 Docosapentaenoic Acid		Docosahexaenoic Acid (DHA)

Chain Length

Long-Chain Fatty Acids (LCFAs) are fats which have between 13 and 21 carbon length chains and include the saturated fats Palmitic Acid, Stearic Acid, and Myristic Acid; monounsaturated fats Oleic Acid; and polyunsaturated fats Linoleic Acid and Alpha-Linolenic Acid (ALA).

Medium-Chain Fatty Acids (MCFAs) are fats which have between 6 and 12 carbon length chains and include Lauric Acid, Capric Acid, Caprylic Acid, and Caproic Acid. The MCFAs are absorbed and transported more easily than LCFAs and are transported straight to the liver to be metabolised[45]. MCFAs have many proposed health benefits including aiding weight loss, increasing insulin sensitivity, and anti-seizure effects[46],[47]. Due to their health benefits, MCFAs are sometimes sold as *MCT oil* supplements (**MCT** = Medium-Chain Triglycerides).

Short-Chain Fatty Acids (SCFAs) are fats which have less than 6 carbon length chains and are produced by the gut microbiota by fermenting prebiotics such as inulin, starch, and fibre[48]. SCFAs are essential for maintaining digestive health and are used in the production of liquids, vitamins, and energy.

Protein

Proteins are the building blocks for every cell in the human body and are composed of Carbon, Hydrogen, Oxygen, and Nitrogen[49]. Just like carbohydrates, protein provides 4 kcal/gram but is rarely used to produce energy. Nitrogen is the most significant part of protein, as a positive Nitrogen balance (i.e. Nitrogen re-synthesis exceeding Nitrogen breakdown), is needed to increase physical performance. Protein contains *Amino Acids* (**Amino** = contains Nitrogen) that form sequences called *Peptides*. Different peptides are needed for fighting infections, building/repairing muscle tissue, transporting oxygen, increasing metabolic reactions and more[50]. Different combinations of peptides form all 22 different amino acids in your body including the *Essential*, *Conditionally Essential*, and *Non-Essential* amino acids.

Essential	Conditionally Essential	Non-Essential
Isoleucine	Arginine	Alanine
Leucine	Cysteine	Asparagine
Lysine	Glutamine	Aspartic Acid
Methionine	Histidine	Citruline
Phenylalanine	Proline	Glutamic Acid
Threonine	Taurine	Glycine
Tryptophan	Tyrosine	Serine
Valine		

Essential Amino Acids

There are 8 essential amino acids including *Isoleucine, Leucine, Lysine, Methionine, Phenylalanine, Threonine, Tryptophan,* and *Valine. Histidine* is an additional essential amino acid during infancy but becomes conditionally essential during adulthood. Each essential amino acid plays an important role within your body.

Leucine is one of 3 *Branched Chain Amino Acids (BCAAs)*. BCAAs get their name because they have a chain branching off one side of their molecular structure. Leucine is the key amino acid for stimulating *Muscle Protein Synthesis (MPS)* and optimising the leucine content of your protein intake is crucial for optimising your performance and hitting your goals[51]. The effect of leucine on MPS is the result of enhanced ribonucleic acid (RNA) translation mediated by increased mTOR phosphorylation[52]. While this is a key component of understanding the importance of increasing leucine content, the main focus should be on selecting high-quality proteins sources. Leucine also helps with blood glucose regulation, wound healing, and producing growth hormones[53].

Isoleucine is another of the BCAAs that aids in muscle protein synthesis and also has anti-catabolic effects[54]. Isoleucine significantly increases glucose uptake and the utilisation of glycogen during exercise and is found in high concentration within muscle tissue[55]. Isoleucine's additional roles include haemoglobin production, energy regulation, and improving immune function[56].

Valine is the last of the BCAAs and with the smallest effect of muscle protein synthesis. No significant benefits have been found for taking valine without leucine and isoleucine, however, more research is needed[57]. Like the other BCAAs, valine is also involved in energy production.

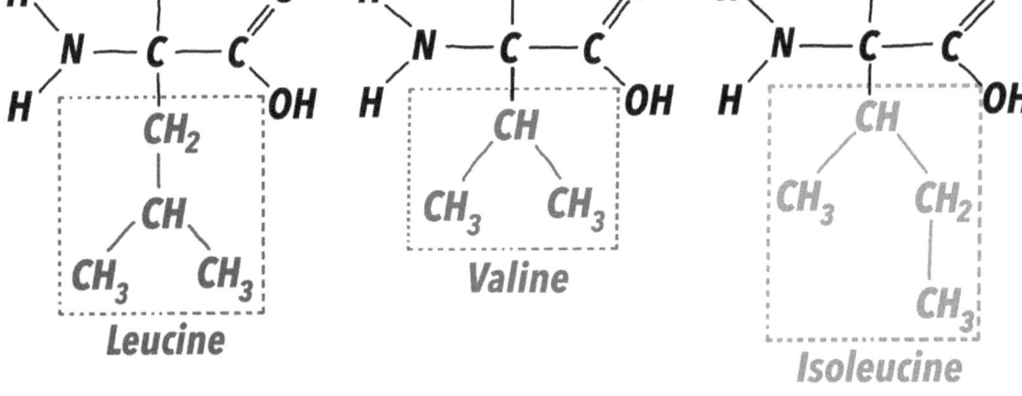

Leucine

Valine

Isoleucine

Phenylalanine is a precursor for the neurotransmitters (**neuro** = relating to nerves or the nervous system) tyrosine, dopamine, epinephrine and norepinephrine[58]. Phenylalanine is involved in the production of other amino acids and plays a key role in the structure and function of different proteins and enzymes.

Threonine is needed to produce structural proteins collagen and elastin which forms your skin and connective tissue. Threonine is also involved in fat metabolism and immune function[59].

Tryptophan is a precursor to the happy hormone serotonin[60]. Low levels of serotonin may cause depression, low mood, low energy, negative thoughts and irritability[61]. Tryptophan is often discussed for its drowsiness effects which be used as a sleep aid by consuming warm milk, turkey, or baked potatoes.

Methionine is needed for tissue growth and aids in the absorption of the trace minerals zinc and selenium[62]. Methionine also aids in detoxifying the body and in metabolism.

Lysine is needed for protein synthesis, hormone production, and enzyme production. Lysine aids in the absorption of the macrominerals calcium and is important for energy production, boosting immune function, and the production of collagen and elastin[63].

Dietary protein is classified as either a *complete protein* (i.e. contains all of the essential amino acids in sufficient amounts) or an *incomplete protein* (i.e. are missing in at least one essential amino acid or have insufficient amounts to be optimal for health or performance). All animal sources of protein (e.g. milk, eggs, meat, and fish) are complete proteins whereas the vast majority of plant proteins are incomplete proteins[64]. Proteins vary in their quality depending on amino acid balance, with the higher the number of essential amino acids, the higher the quality. This will be covered in greater detail in Chapter 5.

Conditionally Essential Amino Acids

There are 7 conditionally essential amino acids including *Arginine*, *Cysteine*, *Glutamine*, *Histidine*, *Proline*, *Taurine*, and *Tyrosine*. These conditionally essential amino acids can be synthesised from the previous 8 essential amino acids but may become essential amino acids if there are insufficient sources of dietary essential amino acids to produce them.

Non-Essential Amino Acids

There are 7 non-essential amino acids including *Alanine*, *Asparagine*, *Aspartic Acid*, *Citruline*, *Glutamic Acid*, *Glycine*, and *Serine*. Non-essential amino acids can be obtained from dietary protein or synthesised within the body in sufficient amounts. Therefore, you do not need to specifically aim to include non-essential amino acids in your diet.

There is a constant exchange of amino acids between the blood, liver, and tissues, with the liver at the centre of this process. The collection of amino acids in these separate areas of the body is known as the *free amino acid pool*. Amino acids are secreted from the liver to meet the demands of rebuilding tissues within the body, whilst also receiving newly obtained amino acids from the diet or those synthesised within the body[65]. This process is kept in perfect balance with any excess being used to meet energy demands, stored as fat, and/or excreted in the urine. There is no dedicated storage for protein itself and so it must be constantly consumed to meet demands. When engaged in regular exercise or trying to change your body composition, this balance between the number of amino acids taken in minus the number of amino acids being used must be kept positive for your desired adaptations to occur.

Practical Applications

The *Acceptable Macronutrient Distribution Range (AMDR)* and *Recommended Daily Allowance (RDA)* for protein, fats, and carbohydrates have been calculated by the Institute of Medicine to maintain a basic level of good health (see table below)[66]. At the most basic level, following these guidelines is suitable for sedentary individuals looking to stay healthy.

	Protein	Fat	Linoleic Acid (Omega-3)	Linolenic Acid (Omega-6)	Carbohydrates	Fibre
AMDR	10 - 35%	25 - 35%	0.6 - 1.2%	5 - 10%	45-65%	
RDA	0.8 g/kg/day		1.6 g/day (Men) 1.1 g/day (Women)	17 g/day (Men) 12 g/day (Women	130 g/day	38 g/day (Men) 25 g/day (Women)

For anyone engaged in regular exercise, trying to improve body composition, or looking for a more bespoke diet to meet their personal preferences, a few more steps are needed to optimise health and performance including specific protein requirements, macronutrient balance, macronutrient periodisation, and portion control.

Protein Requirements

Protein is the most important macronutrient as you require specific amounts relative to your body weight and training goal. Therefore, when planning your diet *you should first calculate your protein requirements then add fats and carbs to reach your caloric needs*. For sedentary adults, consuming 0.8 - 1.0 g/kg/day of protein is sufficient to maintain good health and prevent protein related deficiencies. However, for regularly active individuals, your protein requirements may be much greater depending on your goals and type of exercise you are engaging in. Protein requirements also go up by approx. 1% for every 100 kcal below 2,000 kcal/day and this is part of the reason for recommending a high protein diet when trying to lose excess body fat[67]. The below table provides a guide for your protein intake based upon your activity level or training goal.

Activity Level	Grams of Protein/Kilogram of Bodyweight/Day
Sedentary	0.8 - 1.0
Recreational Exerciser	1.0 - 1.4
Endurance Athletes	1.2 - 1.6
Strength/Power Athletes	1.6 - 2.2
Bodybuilding	1.6 - 2.2
Weight Loss	1.6 - 2.2

Estimating protein needs based solely on exercise type may be too generic therefore it is best to aim for higher values and adjust based upon the length of season, training requirements, body composition etc. A key aspect of increasing protein intake is trying to promote MPS. The role of the essential amino acid leucine is key in attenuating the decrease in nitrogen balance that follows exercise. You can see your protein requirements as trying to raise your leucine levels as quickly and efficiently as possible. To optimise MPS you should *aim to consume between 2-3 g of leucine/meal*. Exercise itself increases MPS however, the timing of your protein intake will be covered in more detail in Chapter 4.

Risks of High Protein Intake

Diets encouraging high protein intake have often been met with concerns over potential harmful effects this may have upon the body, specifically the kidneys. This concern stems from advice given to patients with chronic kidney disease or renal failure who are advised to reduce their protein intake. However, extrapolating this advice to healthy individuals contradicts reviews of the scientific evidence done by the World Health Organization (WHO) and others that showed a lack of evidence linking high protein diets and kidney disease[68]. In fact, research by the International Society of Sports Nutrition (ISSN) showed that diets with extremely high protein intake (~3.4 - 4.4 g/kg/day) reported no harmful effects[69].

Macronutrient Balance

Understanding the role of each of the macronutrients within your body is needed to tailor your macronutrient balance to meet your needs (*macronutrient balance* = the percentage each macronutrient is of your total caloric intake i.e. 50% carbs: 20% protein: 30% fat). As noted earlier, protein is essential to health and performance, so you should first calculate your protein needs using the guide above, then build your fat and carbohydrate intake around this based upon your sport's energy demands and personal preferences. Once you've calculated your needed protein intake you need to convert this into calories to determine how much of your total daily caloric intake is from protein and how much is left for fats and carbohydrates. To help explain we'll use our new friend Mr Semi-Pro.

Mr Semi-Pro

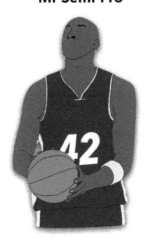

Age: **20**
Height: **193 cm**
Weight: **82.5 kg**
Body Fat: **7%**
Activity: **Basketball 3/w and Resistance Training 4/w**

Mr Semi-Pro's TDEE is 3,616 calories/day and a *protein intake of 165 g/day* (equal to 660 calories). This represents approx. 18% of Mr Semi-Pro's TDEE. This leaves 82% of Mr Semi-Pro's TDEE to be divided between carbohydrates and fat.

Daily Carbohydrate Recommendations for Optimum Performance

The number of carbohydrates you consume should be determined by the intensity and volume of exercise you are engaged in (see table below)[70]. This is based upon ensuring you have enough carbohydrates within your diet to replenish glycogen stores and can maintain your work capacity without drops in performance.

Intensity	Situation	Amount
Light	Low-Intensity or Skill-Based	3 – 5 g/kg/day
Moderate	Moderate-Intensity e.g. 1 hour/day	5 – 7 g/kg/day
High	Endurance Training or Multiple Times/Day e.g. 1-3 hours/day	6 – 10 g/kg/day
Very High	Extreme e.g. Ultra-Marathon, Ironman	10 – 12 g/kg/day

To help explain how these recommendations fit in with your caloric needs and other macronutrients here are a couple of examples using Mr Semi-Pro and Ms Gym Bunny from Chapter 1:

- Mr Semi-Pro is very active playing basketball for multiple hours, 3 times/week and engages in resistance training 4 times/week. Due to the sprint-endurance nature of basketball Mr Semi-Pro needs to eat somewhere between the Moderate and High-Intensity categories to perform at his best. Therefore, a target of 7 g/kg/day would be a good guide. *Mr Semi-Pro would need to eat 578 g of carbohydrates per day (equal to 2,310 calories)* (82.5 kg x 7 g/kg/day = 578 g/day).
- Ms Gym Bunny is your typical regular gym goer and does not need as much carbohydrates as Mr Semi-Pro. Aiming for the low end of the moderate-intensity category (i.e. 5 g/kg/day) means that *Ms Gym Bunny would need to eat 275 g of carbohydrates per day (equal to 1,100 calories)* (55 kg x 5 g/kg/day = 275 g/day).
- In terms of percentage of total caloric intake, this would mean *Mr Semi-Pro is consuming 64%* and *Ms Gym Bunny 49% of their daily calories from carbohydrates*.

Specific carbohydrate recommendations when leading up to an event or fuelling during exercise will be covered in Chapter 4. Once you have calculated your protein and carbohydrates requirements the remainder of calories can be allocated for fat intake using the RDAs above on essential fats to ensure optimum health is achieved because *a healthy athlete is a superior athlete*. You may not want to follow these daily recommended guidelines for carbohydrates indefinitely as there are benefits from alternating between periods of lower and higher carbohydrate intake to improve fat oxidation (**oxidation** = burning) and carbohydrate utilisation which will be covered in the metabolic efficiency section below.

General Health

Macronutrient balance is very simple when it comes to general health, with the balance between fats and carbohydrates mostly determined by personal preference. For example, for a sedentary average height (162 cm) and average weight (60 kg) women, 1,500 calories/day is approximately the correct amount of calories needed to maintain a healthy weight. We know our sedentary woman would need to consume 0.8 - 1.0 g/kg/day of protein, which is equal to 240 calories or 16% of her total daily calories (1.0 x 60 = 60g x 4 kcal/g =

240 kcals). Therefore, our average woman has 1,260 calories which can come from fats or carbs in whichever way is easiest to adhere to. Below are some example macronutrient balance ratios including low-carb, low-fat, and balanced options:

Low-Carb	Balanced	Low-Fat
Protein: 16% - 60g	Protein: 16% - 60g	Protein: 16% - 60g
Carbs: 15% - 56g	Carbs: 50% - 188g	Carbs: 69% - 259g
Fat: 69% - 115g	Fat: 34% - 57g	Fat: 15% - 15g

To ensure the minimum amount of healthy fats are obtained from the diet it is not recommended to follow very low-fat diets like in the example above, long-term. It is also very difficult to adhere to very low-carb diets long-term as shown above so this would not be recommended either. Ultimately, whatever ratio of carbs to fats you choose, try to keep from the extreme ends of the spectrum and select a macronutrient balance you can adhere to consistently to remain in good health.

Does Macronutrient Source Really Matter?

It's worth noting that most foods will contain more than one type of macronutrient which can be both helpful and problematic depending on your macronutrient goals. For example, a cup of *lentils contains approx. 18 grams of protein but also contains 40 grams of carbs*. Therefore, if you are trying to restrict your carbohydrate intake or lose weight this protein source may not be an ideal choice. In this scenario, a good alternative for non-vegans could be eggs, which has the same amount of protein but fewer carbohydrates (*3 large eggs = 18g protein & 1.8g carbs*). The majority of plant-based protein sources are often found in foods which are either high in carbohydrates or fat and can make diet planning a little more difficult, but not impossible. For more examples, check out the Venn diagram opposite.

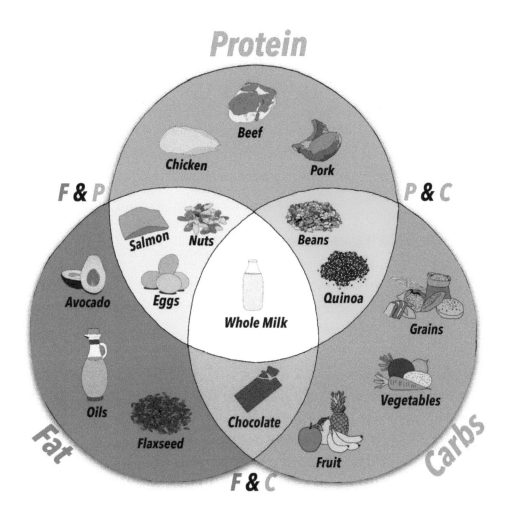

Macronutrient Periodisation

Low carbohydrate/keto diets (see Chapter 7) are a popular option for losing weight and are often advertised as claiming to increase fat oxidation. A key point that should be made however is fat oxidation is higher on low-carb diets because fat intake is higher and what you are providing your body for fuel. On low-fat diets, you burn more carbohydrates because carbohydrate intake is higher and what you are providing your body for fuel. This does not mean you will burn more body fat on a low carb diet and less on a low-fat diet, rather you just burn more of what you consume. A calorie deficit is what determines whether you will burn off or gain body fat. Understanding this is important if you wish to capitalise on improving your body's ability to use different food sources to fuel your exercise demands. By strategically alternating between periods of high and low carbohydrate intake you can improve your body's ability to utilise fat to fuel exercise efforts and to replenish carbohydrate stores more efficiently[71]. In Chapter 1 we discussed the Brooks Crossover Concept where you switch to using carbohydrates to fuel exercise demands once reaching a certain intensity. We also noted this crossover point can be delayed through endurance training. The average adult's glycogen stores equal 1,400 – 2,000 calories which will only last for a couple of hours. If you switch over to burning carbs too early it could result in an inability to finish longer endurance events or not having that final burst of energy for a sprint finish. Signs of poor metabolic efficiency may include the need for regular feeding during endurance work, negative changes in aesthetics and body composition, sluggish behaviour in the afternoon and seeking out caffeine and snacks, slow recovery time or feeling more sore following a new training stimulus. Even in non-endurance sports saving glycogen stores and utilising fat reserves can aid performance and recovery. The ability to capitalise on fat reserves and save glycogen stores is called your *Metabolic Efficiency*.

Metabolic Efficiency

Your metabolic efficiency is determined by approx. 75% diet and 25% exercise. Changes in metabolic efficiency can be achieved in as little as 7 days, although 4 weeks of a dietary change may be better for habit-forming[72]. The more metabolically efficient you become the lower your need for simple sugars to supplement energy demands and therefore, an increased recovery rate and energy levels. The key principles behind optimising your metabolic efficiency are:

- Maintain protein intake throughout.
- Alternate between high-fat/low-carb and high-carb/low-fat.
- Combine protein and fibre to aid digestion.
- Portion guide 1 hand of protein to 1 hand of fibre.
- Better to change long-term diet habits then shifting routines leading up competition i.e. carb-loading.
- Alternate between sleeping low on carbs and/or training low the next morning and sleeping high on carbs and/or training high on carbs.
- And as always KISS (Keep It Simple Stupid).

Portion Control

Counting calories and grams of macronutrients is the most accurate way to track your food intake and is highly recommended for anyone trying to change their body composition or enhance their performance. However, this is not something that needs to be done indefinitely as the ultimate goal is to become an intuitive eater, where you can visually identify the correct portion sizes and food choices without the need for constant monitoring. Strictly tracking your calories and macronutrients for the first few weeks to months of any nutrition plan is the best way to build this skill but it can be helpful to have a backup tracking method or something a little less labour intensive. This is where I would recommend using your hands as a "handy" portion control guide[73].

A "Handy" Portion Control Guide

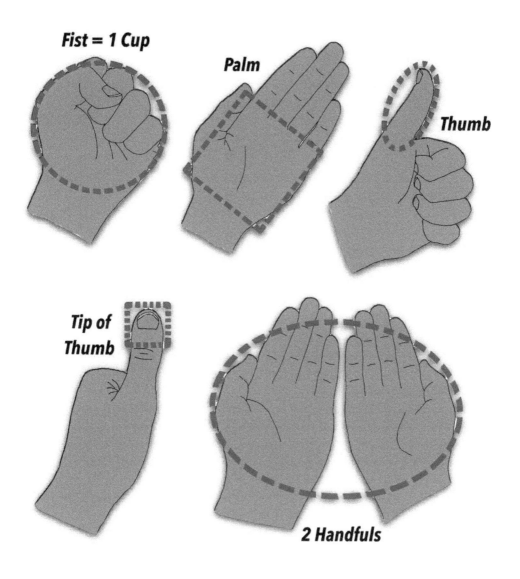

Fist = 1 Cup

Palm

Thumb

Tip of Thumb

2 Handfuls

Fist – Equal to 1 cup and a guide to one portion of fruit, cooked rice, or uncooked pasta.

Palm – Equal to a portion of meat such as chicken or beef.

Thumb – Equal to 2 tablespoons and used to measure portions of dairy or peanut butter.

Tip of Thumb – Equal to 1 teaspoon and used to measure sauces, oils, and butter.

2 Handfuls – Equal to how much fibrous vegetables should be eaten per meal/2-3 portions.

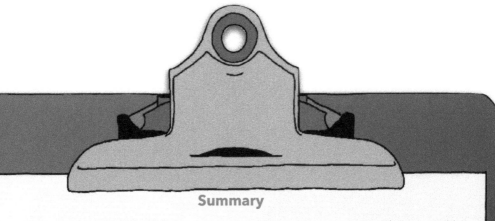

Summary

✓ Macronutrients are **Carbohydrates**, **Fat**, and **Protein**. Carbohydrates are the body's default source of fuel, fats are the body's primary storage form of energy, and protein are the building blocks or every cell in the body.

✓ Carbohydrates are divided into four categories depending on how many sugar units they contain. These four categories are **Monosaccharides** (1 sugar unit), **Disaccharides** (2 sugar units), **Oligosaccharides** (3-9 sugar units), and **Polysaccharides** (10+ sugar units).

✓ Carbohydrates are a non-essential macronutrient that can be created from fat and protein through gluconeogenesis. However, long term carbohydrates restriction leads to changes in fat/carb metabolism that fuels exercise demands.

✓ **Simple Sugars** provide an immediate supply of energy but cause a high insulin response. Whereas **Complex Carbohydrates** slowly release energy and have a much lower insulin response.

✓ Fat is comprised of fatty acids and are divided into **Unsaturated**, **Polyunsaturated**, **Saturated**, and **Trans-Modified** fats, depending upon the amount of double bonds found in each type of fat molecule.

✓ Some fats are needed in the diet as they cannot be created within the body. These fats are called Essential Fatty Acids and include **Linoleic Acid (Omega-3)** and **Linolenic Acid (Omega-6)**.

✓ The human body has a limited capacity to store carbohydrates but an unlimited capacity to store fat.

✓ Protein is made up of **Amino Acids** including 9 **Essential Amino Acids** (must come from diet), 7 **Conditionally Essential Amino Acids** (can be synthesised from other essential amino acids or diet), and 4 **Non-Essential Amino Acids** (created within the body, not required in diet).

✓ 3 of the essential amino acids (Leucine, Isoleucine, and Valine) form a group called **Branched Chain Amino Acids (BCAAs)**, with Leucine playing a key role in **Muscle Protein Synthesis (MPS)**.

✓ All animal proteins sources (e.g. chicken, fish, milk, eggs etc), have all the essential amino acids in sufficient quantities and are known as "**complete protein sources**". All plant sources do not sufficient amounts of all the essential amino acids and are therefore known as "**incomplete protein sources**".

✓ Protein requirements vary depending on your activity levels and training demands ranging from 0.8 – 2.2 g/kg/day. There are no health concerns for high protein intake for healthy individuals. Protein intakes above 2.2g/kg/day have not been shown to provide any additional benefits to performance or health.

✓ Macronutrient balance should start with calculating protein intake and carbohydrates and fats calculated based upon training needs and personal preferences.

✓ Carbohydrate intake should be optimised for performance, based upon training intensity and volume.

✓ Alternating between low-carb and low-fat diet may help improve **Metabolic Efficiency** which has benefits in enhancing recovery, performance, and energy levels.

✓ A simple hand guide to portion control can be used to estimate healthy portion sizes in an attempt to develop a more intuitive style of eating for better long-term diet adherence.

REFERENCES

1 MacLaren, D. and Morton, J. (2012), *Biochemistry for Sport and Exercise Metabolism*, Wiley-Blackwell

2 Antonio, J. et al. (2008), *Essentials of Sports Nutrition and Supplements*, Humana Press

3 Seebohar, B. (2011), *Nutrition Periodization for Athletes: Taking Traditional Sports Nutrition to the Next Level* (2nd Edition). Bull Publishing

4 Oh, R., & Uppaluri, K. R., (2020), *Low Carbohydrate Diet*. [Updated 03/01/2020]. https://www.ncbi.nlm.nih.gov/books/NBK537084/

5 Kahn, S.E., (2003), *The relative contributions of insulin resistance and beta-cell dysfunction to the pathophysiology of Type 2 diabetes*. Diabetologia 46, 3 - 19, https://doi.org/10.1007/s00125-002-1009-0

6 Campbell, C. I., & Spano, M. A., (2011), *NSCA's Guide to Sport and Exercise Nutrition*, Human Kinetics

7 Rizkalla, S.W., (2010), *Health implications of fructose consumption: A review of recent data*. Nutrition & Metabolism 7, 82. https://doi.org/10.1186/1743-7075-7-82

8 Collison, K.S., Saleh, S.M., Bakheet, R.H., Al-Rabiah, R.K., Inglis, A.L., Makhoul, N.J., Maqbool, Z.M., Zaidi, M.Z., Al-Johi, M.A. and Al-Mohanna, F.A. (2009), *Diabetes of the Liver: The Link Between Nonalcoholic Fatty Liver Disease and HFCS-55*. Obesity, 17: 2003-2013. https://doi.org/10.1038/oby.2009.58

9 Mishra, A., Ahmed, K., Froghi, S. and Dasgupta, P. (2015), *Systematic review of the relationship between artificial sweetener consumption and cancer in humans: analysis of 599,741 participants*. The International Journal of Clinical Practice, 69: 1418-1426. https://doi.org/10.1111/ijcp.12703

10 Beards, E., Tuohy, K., & Gibson, G. (2010). *A human volunteer study to assess the impact of confectionery sweeteners on the gut microbiota composition*. British Journal of Nutrition, 104(5), 701-708. https://doi.org/10.1017/S0007114510001078

11 Mattar, R., Mazo, D. F. de C., & Carrilho, F. J. (2012). *Lactose intolerance: Diagnosis, genetic, and clinical factors*. Clinical and Experimental Gastroenterology, 5(1), 113-121. http://dx.doi.org/10.2147/CEG.S32368

12 He, T., Venema, K., Priebe, M.G., Welling, G.W., Brummer, R.-J.M. and Vonk, R.J. (2008), *The role of colonic metabolism in lactose intolerance*. European Journal of Clinical Investigation, 38: 541-547. https://doi.org/10.1111/j.1365-2362.2008.01966.x

13 WhitBread, D., (2020), *Top 10 Foods Highest in Maltose*, Retrieved from https://www.myfooddata.com/articles/high-maltose-foods.php

14 Gibson, G., Probert, H., Loo, J., Rastall, R., & Roberfroid, M. (2004). *Dietary modulation of the human colonic microbiota: Updating the concept of prebiotics*. Nutrition Research Reviews, 17(2), 259-275. https://doi.org/10.1079/NRR200479

15 Roberfroid, M. B., (2007), *Inulin-Type Fructans: Functional Food Ingredients*, The Journal of Nutrition, 137(11), 2493S–2502S, https://doi.org/10.1093/jn/137.11.2493S

16 Carlson, J. L., Erickson, J. M., Lloyd, B. B., & Slavin, J. L. (2018). *Health Effects and Sources of Prebiotic Dietary Fiber*. Current developments in nutrition, 2(3), nzy005. https://doi.org/10.1093/cdn/nzy005

17 Tortora, G. J. & Derrickson, B., (2017), *Principles of Anatomy & Physiology*, Wiley & Sons Inc.

18 Smith Rockwell, M., Walberg Rankin, J., & Dixon, H., (2003), *Effects of Muscle Glycogen on Performance of Repeated Sprints and Mechanisms of Fatigue*, 13(1), 1-14, https://doi.org/10.1123/ijsnem.13.1.1

19 Zou, W., Yu, L., Liu, X., Chen, L., Zhang, X., Qiao, D., and Zhang, R., (2012), *Effects of amylose/amylopectin ratio on starch-based superabsorbent polymers*, Carbohydrate Polymers, 87(2), 1583-1588, https://doi.org/10.1016/j.carbpol.2011.09.060

20 Dhingra, D., Michael, M., and Rajput, H. (2012), *Dietary fibre in foods: a review*. Journal of Food Science Technology **49,** 255–266, https://doi.org/10.1007/s13197-011-0365-5

21 Pereira, M. A., O'Reilly, E., Augustsson, K., Fraser, G. E., Goldbourt, U., Heitmann, B. L., Hallmans, G., Knekt, P., Liu, S., Pietinen, P., Spiegelman, D., Stevens, J., Virtamo, J., Willett, W. C., and Ascherio, A., (2004), *Dietary Fiber and Risk of Coronary Heart Disease: A Pooled Analysis of Cohort Studies*, Archives of Internal Medicine, 164(4), 370-376, https://doi.org/10.1001/archinte.164.4.370

22 Sebely, P., Khossousi, A., Binns, C., Dhaliwal, S., and Ellis, V., (2011). *The effect of a fibre supplement compared to a healthy diet on body composition, lipids, glucose, insulin and other metabolic syndrome risk factors in overweight and obese individuals*. British Journal of Nutrition, 105(1), 90-100, https://doi.org/10.1017/S0007114510003132

23 Brouns. F., Theuwissen, E., Adam, A., Bell, M., Berger, A., and Mensink, R. P., (2012), *Cholesterol-lowering properties of different pectin types in mildly hyper-cholesterolemic men and women*. European Journal of Clinical Nutrition, 66(5):591-9, https://doi.org/10.1038/ejcn.2011.208

24 Chen, J., & Raymond, K. (2008). *Beta-glucans in the treatment of diabetes and associated cardiovascular risks*. Vascular health and risk management, 4(6), 1265–1272. https://doi.org/10.2147/vhrm.s3803

25 Akramiene, D., Kondrotas, A., Didziapetriene, J., and Kevelaitis, E., (2007), *Effects of beta-glucans on the immune system*, Medicina (Kaunas), 43(8), 597-606, https://doi.org/10.3390/medicina43080076

26 Mudgil, D., Barak, S., PAtel, and Shah, N., (2018), *Partially hydrolyzed guar gum as a potential prebiotic source*, International Journal of Biological Macromolecules, 112, 207-210, https://doi.org/10.1016/j.ijbiomac.2018.01.164

27 Butt, M. S., Shahzadi, N., Sharif, M. K., & Nasir, M., (2007) *Guar Gum: A Miracle Therapy for Hypercholesterolemia, Hyperglycemia and Obesity*, Critical Reviews in Food Science and Nutrition, 47(4), 389-396, https://doi.org/10.1080/10408390600846267

28 Singh, D. K. & Ray, A. R., (2000), *Biomedical Applications of Chitin, Chitosan, and Their Derivatives*, Journal of Macromolecular Science, Part C, 40(1), 69-83, https://doi.org/10.1081/MC-100100579

29 MacLaren, D. and Morton, J. (2012), *Biochemistry for Sport and Exercise Metabolism*, Wiley-Blackwell

30 Tremblay, A. (2004), *Dietary Fat and Body Weight Set Point*, Nutrition Reviews, 62(2), S75–S77, https://doi.org/10.1111/j.1753-4887.2004.tb00092.x

31 NIH, National Institute of General Medical Sciences (NIGMS). (2013). *The biology of fats in the body*. ScienceDaily. Retrieved from www.sciencedaily.com/releases/2013/04/130423102127.htm

32 Libby, P., Ridker, P. M., and Maseri, A., (2002), *Inflammation and Atherosclerosis*, Circulation, 105, 1135-1143, https://doi.org/10.1161/hc0902.104353

33 Mensink, R. P., (2005), *Effects of stearic acid on plasma lipid and lipoproteins in humans*. Lipids 40, 1201–1205, https://doi.org/10.1007/s11745-005-1486-x

34 Kien, C. L., Bunn, J. Y., Stevens, R., Bain, J., Ikayeva, O., Crain, K., Koves, T. R., and Muoio, D. M., (2014), *Dietary intake of palmitate and oleate has broad impact on systemic and tissue lipid profiles in humans*, The American Journal of Clinical Nutrition, 99(3), 436-445, https://doi.org/10.3945/ajcn.113.070557

35 Hunter, J. E., Zhang, J. and Kris-Etherton, P. M., (2010), *Cardiovascular disease risk of dietary stearic acid compared with trans, other saturated, and unsaturated fatty acids: a systematic review*, The American Journal of Clinical Nutrition, 91(1), 46–63, https://doi.org/10.3945/ajcn.2009.27661

36 Mensik, R. P., Zock, P. L., Kester, A. D. and Katan, M. B., (2003), *Effects of dietary fatty acids and carbohydrates on the ratio of serum total to HDL cholesterol and on serum lipids and apolipoproteins: a meta-analysis of 60 controlled trials*. The American Journal of Clinical Nutrition, 77(5), 1146-1155, https://doi.org/10.1093/ajcn/77.5.1146

37 Temme, E. H., Mensink, R. P. and Hornstra, G., (1996), *Comparison of the effects of diets enriched in lauric, palmitic, or oleic acids on serum lipids and lipoproteins in healthy women and men*, The American Journal of Clinical Nutrition, 63(6), 897-903, https://doi.org/10.1093/ajcn/63.6.897

38 Guasch-Ferré, M., Hu, F.B., Martínez-González, M.A., Fitó, M., Bulló, M., Estruch, R., Ros, E., Corella, D., Recondo, J., Gómez-Gracia, E., Fiol, M., Lapetra, J., Serra-Majem, L., Muñoz, M. A., Pintó, X., Lamuela-Raventós, R. M., Basora, J., Buil-Cosiales, P., Sorlí, J. V., Ruiz-Gutiérrez, V., Martínez, J. A. and Salas-Salvadó. J., (2014), *Olive oil intake and risk of cardiovascular disease and mortality in the PREDIMED Study*. BMC Medicine, **12**, 78 (2014). https://doi.org/10.1186/1741-7015-12-78

39 Wanders, A. J., Zock, P. L. and Brouwer, I.A. (2017), *Trans Fat Intake and Its Dietary Sources in General Populations Worldwide: A Systematic Review*. Nutrients, 9, 840. https://doi.org/10.3390/nu9080840

40 National Institutes of Health, (2019), *Omega-3 Fatty Acids: Fact Sheet for Health Professionals*, Retrieved from https://ods.od.nih.gov/factsheets/Omega3FattyAcids-HealthProfessional/

41 Simopoulos, A. P., (2008), *The importance of the omega-6/omega-3 fatty acid ratio in cardiovascular disease and other chronic diseases*, Experimental Biology and Medicine, 233(6), 674-688, https://doi.org/10.3181/0711-MR-311

42 Dinan, T., Siggins, L., Scully, P., O'Brien, S., Ross, P. and Stanton, C., (2009), *Investigating the inflammatory phenotype of major depression: Focus on cytokines and polyunsaturated fatty acids*, Journal of Psychiatric Research, 43(4), 471-476, https://doi.org/10.1016/j.jpsychires.2008.06.003

43 Calder, P. C., (2006), *n-3 polyunsaturated fatty acids, inflammation, and inflammatory diseases*, The American Journal of Clinical Nutrition, 83(6), 1505S-1519S, https://doi.org/10.1093/ajcn/83.6.1505S

44 Gammone, M. A., Riccioni, G., Parrinello, G. and D'Orazio, N., (2019), *Omega-3 Polyunsaturated Fatty Acids: Benefits and Endpoints in Sport*, Nutrients, 11(1), 46, https://doi.org/10.3390/nu11010046

45 Marten, B., Pfeuffer, M. and Schrezenmeir, J., (2006), *Medium-chain triglycerides*, International Dairy Journal, 16(11), 1374-1382, https://doi.org/10.1016/j.idairyj.2006.06.015

46 Liu, Y. M. & Wang, H. S., (2013), *Medium-chain triglyceride ketogenic diet, an effective treatment for drug-resistant epilepsy and a comparison with other ketogenic diets*. Biomedical Journal, 36(1):9-15. https://doi.org/10.4103/2319-4170.107154

47 Examine.com, (2020), *Medium-chain triglycerides*, Retrieved from: https://examine.com/supplements/mcts/

48 den Besten, G., van Eunen, K., Groen, A. K., Venema, K., Reijngoud, D-J. and Bakker, B. M., (2013), *The role of short-chain fatty acids in the interplay between diet, gut microbiota, and host energy metabolism*, Journal of Lipid Research, 54(9), 2325-2340, https://doi.org/https://dx.doi.org/10.1194%2Fjlr.R036012

49 MacLaren, D. and Morton, J. (2012), *Biochemistry for Sport and Exercise Metabolism*, Wiley-Blackwell

50 Berg, J. M., Tymoczko, J. L. Gatto, Jr., G. J. and Stryer, L., (2015), *Biochemistry*, 8th Edition, Palgrave Macmillan

51 Reitelseder, S., Agergaard, J., Doessing, S., Helmark, I. C., Lund, P., Kristensen, N. B., Frystyk, J., Flyvbjerg, A., Schjerling, P., van Hall, G., Kjaer, M. and Holm, L., (2011), *Whey and casein labeled with l-[1-13C]leucine and muscle protein synthesis: effect of resistance exercise and protein ingestion*, American Journal of Physiology-Endocrinology and Metabolism, 300(1), E231-E242, https://doi.org/10.1152/ajpendo.00513.2010

52 Pasiakos, S. M. (2012), *Exercise and amino acid anabolic cell signaling and the regulation of skeletal muscle mass*. Nutrients, 4, 740-758, https://doi.org/10.3390/nu4070740

53 Duan, Y., Li, F., Li, Y., Tang, Y., Kong, X., Feng, Z., Anthony, T. G., Watford, M., Hou, Y., Wu, G. and Yin, Y., (2016), *The role of leucine and its metabolites in protein and energy metabolism*. Amino Acids 48, 41–51. https://doi.org/10.1007/s00726-015-2067-1

54 Zhang, S., Zeng, X., Ren, M. *et al.* (2017), *Novel metabolic and physiological functions of branched chain amino acids: a review*. Journal of Animal Science and Biotechnology, 8, 10, https://doi.org/10.1186/s40104-016-0139-z

55 Blomstrand, E. & Saltin, B., (1999), *Effect of muscle glycogen on glucose, lactate and amino acid metabolism during exercise and recovery in human subjects*, The Journal of Physiology, 1(514), 293-302, https://dx.doi.org/10.1111%2Fj.1469-7793.1999.293af.x

56 National Library of Medicine, (2020), *l-Isoleucine*, Retrieved from https://pubchem.ncbi.nlm.nih.gov/compound/l-isoleucine

57 National Library of Medicine, (2020), *Valine*, Retrieved from https://pubchem.ncbi.nlm.nih.gov/compound/L-valine

58 Fernstrom, J. D. & Fernstrom, M. H., (2007), *Tyrosine, Phenylalanine, and Catecholamine Synthesis and Function in the Brain*, The Journal of Nutrition, 137(6), 1539S–1547S, https://doi.org/10.1093/jn/137.6.1539S

59 National Library of Medicine, (2020), *L-Threonine*, Retrieved from https://pubchem.ncbi.nlm.nih.gov/compound/threonine

60 Jenkins, T. A., Nguyen, J. C. D., Polglaze, K. E. and Bertrand, P. P., (2016), *Influence of Tryptophan and Serotonin on Mood and Cognition with a Possible Role of the Gut-Brain Axis*, Nutrients, 8(1), 56, https://dx.doi.org/10.3390%2Fnu8010056

61 Young, S. N., (2013), *Acute tryptophan depletion in humans: a review of theoretical, practical and ethical aspects*, Journal of Psychiatry & Neuroscience, 38(5), 294-305, https://dx.doi.org/10.1503%2Fjpn.120209

62 National Library of Medicine, (2020), *Methionine*, Retrieved from https://pubchem.ncbi.nlm.nih.gov/compound/L-methionine

63 National Library of Medicine, (2020), *Lysine*, Retrieved from https://pubchem.ncbi.nlm.nih.gov/compound/L-lysine

64 Hoffman, J. R. & Falvo, M. J., (2005), *Protein - Which is Best?*, Journal of Sports Science & Medicine, 3(3), 118-130, https://www.ncbi.nlm.nih.gov/pmc/articles/PMC3905294/#__ffn_sectitle

65 Pitkänen, H. T., Nykänen, T., Knuutinen, J., Lahti, K., Keinänen, O., Alen, M., Komi, P. V., Mero, A. A., (2003), *Free Amino Acid Pool and Muscle Protein Balance after Resistance Exercise*, Medicine & Science in Sports & Exercise, 35(5), 784-792, https://doi.org/10.1249/01.MSS.0000064934.51751.F9

66 Institute of Medicine, (2005), *Dietary Reference Intakes for Energy, Carbohydrate, Fiber, Fat, Fatty Acids, Cholesterol, Protein, and Amino Acids*, The National Academies Press, https://www.nal.usda.gov/sites/default/files/fnic_uploads/energy_full_report.pdf

67 Kraemer, WJ, Fleck, SJ, and Deschenes, M. (1988), *A review: Factors in exercise prescription of resistance training*. NSCA Journal 110, 36-41, https://journals.lww.com/nsca-scj/Citation/1988/10000/EXERCISE_PHYSIOLOGY_CORNER__A_ReviewFactors_in.6.aspx

68 FAO/WHO/UNU, (2002), *Protein and amino acid requirements in human nutrition*. Geneva: World Health Organization; 2002(Series Editor): Who technical report series

69 Antonio, J., Ellerbroek, A., Silver, T., Vargas, L., Tamayo, A., Buehn, R., Peacock, C. A., (2016), *A high protein diet has no harmful effects: a one-year crossover study in resistance-trained males*. Journal of Nutrition and Metabolism, 2016:9104792, https://dx.doi.org/10.1155%2F2016%2F9104792

70 Burke, L., Hawley, J., Wong, S. & Jeukendrup, A., (2011). *Carbohydrates for training and competition*. Journal of sports sciences. 29(1). S17-S27. https://doi.org10.1080/02640414.2011.585473

[71] Burke, L. M., (2010), *Fueling strategies to optimize performance: training high or training low?*, Scandinavian Journal of Medicine & Science in Sports, 20(S2), https://doi.org/10.1111/j.1600-0838.2010.01185.x

[72] Rowlands, D. S. & Hopkins, W. G., (2002), *Effects of high-fat and high-carbohydrate diets on metabolism and performance in cycling.* Metabolism 51(6): 678-690, https://doi.org/10.1053/meta.2002.32723

[73] Precision Nutrition, (2020), *Forget Calorie Counting*, Retrieved from https://www.precisionnutrition.com/calorie-control-guide

3

MICRONUTRIENTS & HYDRATION

What are micronutrients and how much water is enough?

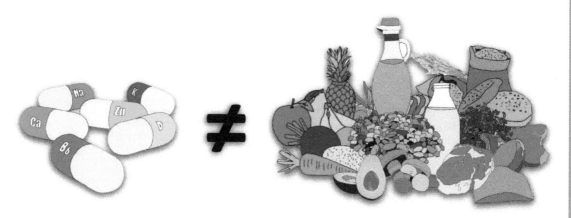

Micronutrients (***micro*** = small) are substances required in trace amounts to support normal physiological function and health[1]. However, while deficiencies in micronutrients can impair health and performance, excess amounts of some micronutrients can also have a harmful effect. Micronutrients divide into 2 categories - *Vitamins* and *Minerals*. There are 13 different vitamins and 16 different minerals that serve unique purposes within the body. Physical activity may increase your micronutrient requirements; however, there is little evidence into the potential benefits of supplementing most vitamins and minerals to improve performance.

Vitamins

For a compound to be classified as a vitamin, it must be clear that insufficient amounts will be detrimental to health and that the restoration of the missing compound will prevent or cure symptoms[2]. Vitamins divide into 2 categories, *Water-Soluble* and *Fat-Soluble* - based upon how each vitamin behaves within the body. Fat-soluble vitamins are absorbed in fat globules called *Chylomicrons* which travel around the body until used, or are stored in body fat for later use. Because these vitamins are stored in body fat, it is possible to have dangerous levels of these vitamins within the body called *hypervitaminosis*[3]. Water-soluble vitamins are absorbed in water and unused water-soluble vitamins are excreted in the urine. However, it is still possible to consume excess amounts of water-soluble vitamins, although this is much more difficult when getting your vitamins from natural sources and not high-dose supplements.

Water-Soluble Vitamins

Thiamine (Vitamin B1)

Found in the body as free absorbable Thiamine or as the molecules *Thiamine Monophosphate (TMP)*, *Thiamine Triphosphate (TTP)*, and *Thiamine Pyrophosphate (TPP)*. Of the Thiamine in the body 10% is TMP, 80% is TPP, and 10% is TTP. Thiamine is involved in muscle contraction, the sending of nerve signals, and the conversion of carbohydrates into energy. Deficiencies in Thiamine can lead to Beriberi or Wernicke-Korsakoff syndrome[4]. The Recommended Daily Allowance (RDA) for Thiamine is **1.2 mg/day (men)**, or **1.1 mg/day (women)**.

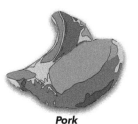

Pork

Salmon

Flaxseed

Riboflavin (Vitamin B2)

Riboflavin forms an essential part of two *Coenzymes* (compounds that aid in biochemical reactions). These two coenzymes are *Flavin Mononucleotide (FMN)* and *Flavin Adenine Dinucleotide (FAD)*. Riboflavins are needed for the metabolism of macronutrients and are involved in growth and red blood cell production. Deficiencies in Riboflavin can lead to sore throats, cracks and sores on the lips and mouth, and redness and swelling of the mouth and throat[5]. The RDA for Riboflavin is **1.3 mg/day (men)**, or **1.1 mg/day (women)**.

Beef

Milk

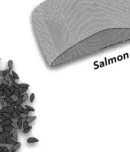

Salmon

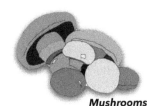

Mushrooms

Niacin (Vitamin B3)

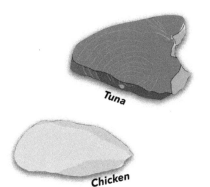
Tuna

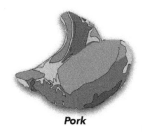
Chicken

Within the body, Niacin is utilised in four different forms: *Nicotinic Acid*, *Nicotinamide*, *Nicotinamide Adenine Dinucleotide (NAD)*, and *Nicotinamide Adenine Dinucleotide Phosphate (NADP)*. NAD and NADP are coenzymes required by around 200 different enzymes, needed for the breakdown of all macronutrients as well as the synthesis of fatty acids and cholesterol. Niacin also helps the digestive system, nerves, and skin to function properly. Niacin can be synthesised within the body from the essential amino acid tryptophan. However, Niacin is classified as a vitamin due to deficiencies in Niacin leading to Pellagra, or in minor cases irritability, poor concentration, anxiety, fatigue, and depression[6]. The RDA for Niacin is **16 mg/day (men)**, or **14 mg/day (women)**.

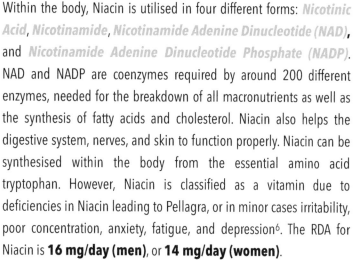
Pork

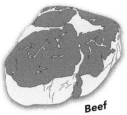
Beef

Pantothenic Acid (Vitamin B5)

Primarily serves as a component of *Coenzyme A (CoA)*, which is vital to several biochemical reactions including the production of the energy molecule *Adenosine Triphosphate (ATP)* from macronutrients. Pantothenic Acid also aids in the production of hormones and cholesterol. Deficiencies in Pantothenic Acid can cause fatigue, insomnia, depression, irritability, burning feet, and chest infections[7]. The RDA for Pantothenic Acid is **5 mg/day (men & women)**.

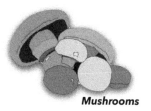
Mushrooms

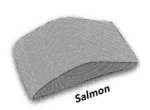
Salmon

Avocados

Vitamin B6

Found in the body in 6 different forms: *Pyridoxal*, *Pyridoxine*, *Pyridoxamine*, *Pyridoxal 5'-Phosphate (PLP)*, *Pyridoxine 5'-Phosphate*, and *Pyridoxamine 5'- Phosphate*. PLP is a coenzyme that is important in the release of muscle glycogen for energy production and gluconeogenesis. Vitamin B6 is also involved in making antibodies, normal nerve function, making haemoglobin, and regulating blood sugar levels. Vitamin B6 deficiency can cause dermatitis, depression, confusion, anaemia, and convulsions. Excess Vitamin B6 can lead to nerve damage in the arms and legs[8]. The RDA for Vitamin B6 is **1.3 mg/day (men & women)**.

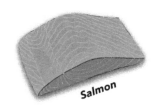

Salmon

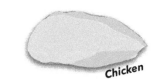

Chicken

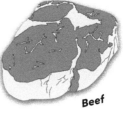

Beef

Biotin (Vitamin B7)

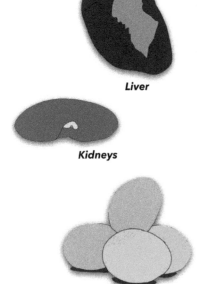

Liver

Kidneys

Attaches to 4 different enzymes *Acetyl-CoA Carboxylase*, *Pyruvate Carboxylase*, *Methylcrotonyl-CoA Carboxylase*, and *Propionyl-CoA Carboxylase*. Acetyl-CoA Carboxylase is needed to produce fatty acids; Pyruvate Carboxylase is important in gluconeogenesis; Methylcrotonyl-CoA Carboxylase is needed to metabolise Leucine (one of the 9 essential amino acids), and Propionyl-CoA Carboxylase is needed in the metabolism of various amino acids, fatty acids, and cholesterol. Biotin deficiency can cause dermatitis, hair loss, hallucinations, numbness in the extremities, and ataxia[9]. The RDA for Biotin is **30 μg/day (men & women)** (*μg* = micrograms, 1 microgram = 0.001 milligram).

Egg Yolks

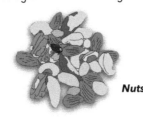

Nuts

54

Folate (Vitamin B9)

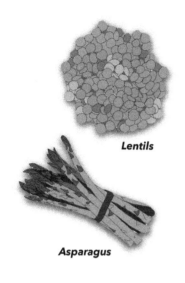

Lentils

Also known as *Folic Acid* (a man-made version of folate), Folate is essential in Deoxyribonucleic Acid (DNA) production, helps in tissue growth and function, works with Vitamin B12 and Vitamin C to breakdown, use, and create new proteins, and also helps in forming new red blood cells. Deficiencies in folate can lead to anaemia[10]. The RDA for Folate is **400 µg/day (men & women)**.

Asparagus

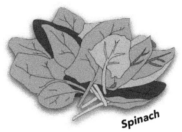

Spinach

Cobalamin (Vitamin B12)

Vitamin B12 is the largest and most complex vitamin. Vitamin B12 contains cobalt and this is where the name Cobalamin comes from. Vitamin B12 forms part of *Methylcobalamin* and *5-deoxyadenosyl Cobalamin*. Methylcobalamin is required for protein metabolism, specifically in the synthesis of Methionine (another of the essential amino acids). 5-deoxyadenosyl Cobalamin is involved in the conversion of coenzymes needed for energy production from fats and proteins. Low-level deficiencies in B12 can lead to anaemia, fatigue, depression, and mania whereas long term deficiency can lead to permanent brain and central nervous system damage[11]. The RDA for Vitamin B12 is **2.4 µg/day (men & women)**.

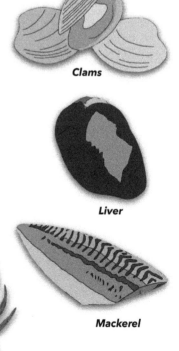

Clams

Liver

Mackerel

Crab

Vitamin C

Also called *Ascorbic Acid*, Vitamin C is essential to produce collagen and is a key component of tendons, ligaments, bones, and blood vessels. Vitamin C is also involved in the production of Carnitine, a fatty acid transport molecule that transports fats to the *Mitochondria* (energy cells) to use as fuel (once converted into ATP). Finally, the most well know use of Vitamin C is as an anti-oxidant, protecting against the effects of free radicals (loose electrons that can trigger cell mutations and disease). Vitamin C deficiency can lead to scurvy which includes symptoms of internal bleeding, gingivitis, poor wound healing, fatigue and depression[12]. Sailors used to have high outbreaks of scurvy due to long voyages without access to fresh fruit[13]. The RDA for Vitamin C is **90 mg/day (men)** or **75 mg/day (women)**.

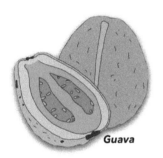
Guava

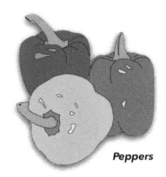
Peppers

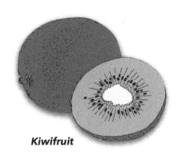
Kiwifruit

What happened to the missing B Vitamins and what are Energy Vitamins?

A few other compounds have been previously labelled as vitamins and given a letter and/or number amongst the other vitamins (e.g. Adenine, previously known as Vitamin B4). However, these former vitamins have since lost their vitamin status, as their role within the body is now better understood. The important thing is to focus on the remaining 13 (true) vitamins.

B Vitamins are sometimes referred to as "energy vitamins" as they are all involved (in one way or another), in the production of energy (ATP) within the body. However, it is important to understand that B vitamins do not provide energy directly, rather they aid in the production of energy from other sources. Therefore, taking B vitamin supplements with an unbalanced and low diversity diet could still cause low energy levels and poor performance. B vitamin supplementation is particularly important to vegetarians who lack good non-fortified sources of B6 & B12.

Fat-Soluble Vitamins

Vitamin A

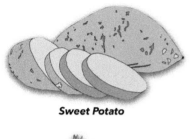

Sweet Potato

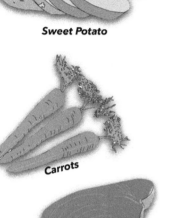

Carrots

Vitamin A includes a group of compounds called *Retinoids*, which include *Retinol*, *Retinal*, and *Retinoic Acid*. Retinol is part of the protein Rhodopsin, which absorbs light in the eye and therefore Vitamin A is essential in maintaining healthy sight. Vitamin A also plays a role in the normal functioning of the lungs, heart, kidneys, and other organs, as well as contributing to immune function, cellular communication, and reproduction. Vitamin A deficiency can lead to blindness and an increased amount of viral infections. Excess consumption of Vitamin A can cause jaundice (i.e. yellowing of the skin), nausea, irritability and hair loss[14]. The RDA for Vitamin A is **900 µg/day (men)**, or **700 µg/day (women)**.

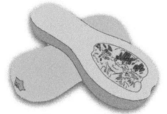

Tuna

Butternut Squash

Vitamin D

Vitamin D is found not only in foods but can also be created within the body when a large amount of skin (e.g. the face and arms or more), is exposed to ultraviolet light (i.e. sunlight), specifically UVB. Vitamin D is inactive in its obtained form and must be converted in the body into more active forms. The most significant active form in the body is *Cholecalciferol (D3)*. Vitamin D aids in the absorption of minerals (e.g. Calcium, Magnesium, and Phosphate), and is needed for healthy bone remodelling. You also need Vitamin D to prevent bones from becoming thin and brittle, as well as in regulating cell growth, neuromuscular and immune system function, and the reduction of inflammation. As Vitamin D can be obtained from non-food sources it is not strictly speaking a true vitamin. However, Vitamin D has maintained its vitamin status as deficiency may lead to Rickets, a weakened immune system, an increased risk for cancer, and poor hair growth. Excess intake of Vitamin D can cause excess Calcium absorption, which increases the

UVB Sunlight

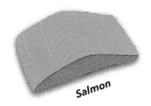

Salmon

risk of cardiovascular disease through hardening of the arteries, as well as an increase in kidney stones[15]. The RDA for Vitamin D is **15 µg/day (men & women)**, although during the summer months most people will get the majority of their needed Vitamin D from sun exposure alone and not just their diet.

Vitamin E

Vitamin E is a name given to a group of anti-oxidants including *Tocopherols* and *Tocotrienols*. Tocopherols and Tocotrienols are further divided into alpha (α), beta (β), gamma (γ), and delta (δ) forms (α, β, γ & δ are the first 4 letters of the Greek alphabet. Science, maths, and technology often use the Greek alphabet when classifying things). α-Tocopherol is the most active form of Vitamin E and is a powerful anti-oxidant, protecting against potential disease-causing free radicals, particularly during the breakdown of fats for use as energy. Vitamin E deficiency can cause poor nerve transmission and muscle weakness whereas excess amounts of Vitamin E can lead to excessive bleeding[16]. The RDA for Vitamin E is **15 mg/day (men & women)**.

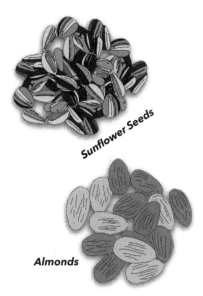

Sunflower Seeds

Almonds

Vitamin K

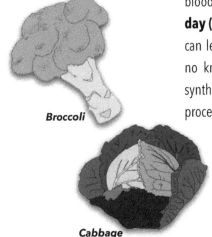

Kale

Broccoli

Vitamin K has two naturally occurring forms: *Phylloquinone* (Vitamin K1) and *Menaquinone-n* (Vitamin K2). Phylloquinone found in plant sources, is the primary dietary form of Vitamin K, whereas Menaquinone-n comes from bacteria in the gut. You need Vitamin K in your diet for healthy bone remodelling and forming blood clots for healing wounds[17]. The RDA for Vitamin K is **120 µg/day (men)**, or **90 µg/day (women)**. Vitamin K deficiency is rare but can lead to excessive bleeding due to poor clotting ability. There are no known concerns over high Vitamin K intake. As Vitamin K2 is synthesised by the gut bacteria, it is important to eat a diverse, low processed food diet to facilitate a healthy gut microbiome[18].

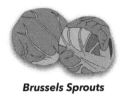

Brussels Sprouts

Cabbage

Minerals

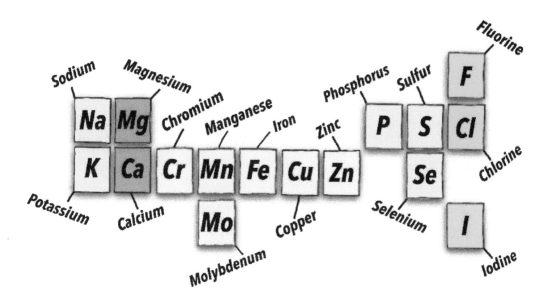

Minerals are inorganic substances (i.e. not from living organisms), and are involved in several functions within the body. Some minerals are needed in larger amounts (*Macrominerals*) and some in smaller amounts (*Trace Minerals*). However, despite some minerals being needed in smaller amounts than others, all minerals are essential for healthy development and performance. Minerals are absorbed a lot more efficiently from the diet than from supplements. A person deficient in one mineral or vitamin may often be deficient in multiple minerals of vitamins. When this happens, analysing the diet is vital, as changes to your diet will be more effective at correcting deficiencies than supplementation alone.

"What you find at the end of your fork is more powerful than anything you'll find at the bottom of a pill bottle" [19]

Macrominerals

Calcium

Calcium is the most abundant mineral in the body with 99% of Calcium within the body stored in the bones and teeth. Calcium is needed for the contraction and dilation of the blood vessels, hormonal secretion, muscle function, and sending signals around the body (e.g. when a nerve impulse tells a muscle to contract)[20]. Calcium is also extremely important to maintain bone strength. Without sufficient amounts of Calcium, there is a significant increase in the risk of developing *Osteoporosis* (a condition characterised by low bone density and increased fracture risk). As the bones are under constant reconstruction, a constant supply of dietary Calcium is needed to ensure that the amount of Calcium available to support new building by the *Osteoblasts* is greater than the amount broken down by the *Osteoclasts*[21]. Vitamin D is vital to the absorption of Calcium and therefore several high Calcium food sources are often fortified with Vitamin D to support Calcium bioavailability (more on this later). The RDA for Calcium is **1,000 mg/day (men & women)**. Calcium requirements increase a little with age with men >70 years old and women >50 years old requiring 1,200 mg/day.

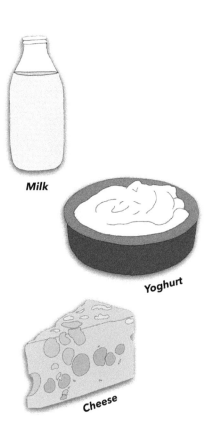

Milk

Yoghurt

Cheese

Chloride

Chloride is needed for fluid regulation, particularly by balancing electrolytes (more on this later). Chloride interacts with several other minerals within the body namely Sodium and Potassium and is important in regulating the pH of the stomach acid. Deficiencies in Chloride can cause sweating, diarrhoea, and vomiting, whereas excess Chloride can cause increases in blood pressure and can cause complications for patients with congestive heart failure[22]. The RDA for Chloride is **2.3 g/day (men & women)**, decreasing to 2.0 g/day for men & women over 50 years old.

Salt

Kelp (Seaweed)

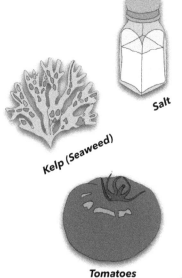

Tomatoes

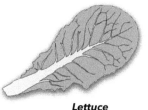

Lettuce

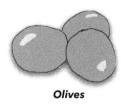

Olives

Magnesium

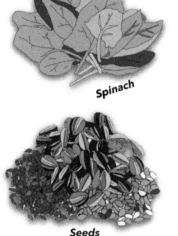

Spinach

Seeds

Magnesium is needed by over 300 biochemical reactions in the body and helps to maintain normal muscle and nerve function, supports the immune system, helps regulate heart rate, maintains bone strength, helps regulate blood glucose levels and assists in energy production and protein synthesis. Deficiencies in magnesium can cause muscle weakness, sleepiness, irregular heart rhythms, and/or hyperexcitability. However, severe deficiencies in magnesium are rare. Excess magnesium can cause diarrhoea where the body attempts to eliminate the build-up[23]. The RDA for Magnesium is **420 mg/day (men)**, or **320 mg/day (women)**.

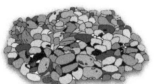

Beans

Sodium

Sodium has received a lot of attention and is often branded as a must avoid nutrient. However, Sodium is needed to regulate blood pressure, it helps in conducting nerve signals, maintains fluid balance, and maintain a healthy heart rate[24]. Deficiencies in Sodium are more common in athletes due to possible excessive water consumption or increased Sodium loss during exercise from heavy sweating. Individuals on "juicing fasts" are also likely to be deficient in Sodium as well as many more nutrients due to this unhealthy practice. Excess Sodium has been linked to increased risk of cardiovascular disease, however, this link is not independent of excess weight and overall poor-quality diet. Therefore, overweight individuals would be better served improving their overall diet quality and losing weight, rather than focusing on the reduction of one micronutrient. The RDA for Sodium is **1.5 g/day (men & women)**, however, some research has shown that optimum balance for healthy and active individuals may be closer to 3.0 - 4.0 g/day of salt[25].

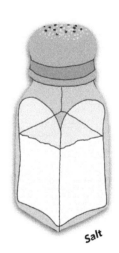

Salt

Potassium

Potassium is another essential nutrient needed to maintain fluid balance within the body. Potassium serves a vital function in maintaining healthy nerve conduction as well as energy metabolism, cellular growth, and glycogenesis. Deficiencies in potassium can lead to several serious conditions including decreased cardiac output, high blood pressure, fatigue, and possible complications in the respiratory, renal, cardiovascular, and endocrine systems. Excess potassium is very rare but can lead to weakness, paralysis, and heart palpitations[26]. The RDA for Potassium is **4.7 g/day (men & women)**.

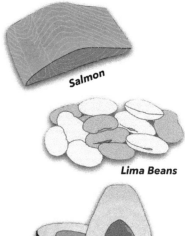
Salmon

Lima Beans

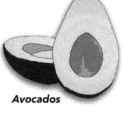
Avocados

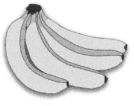
Bananas

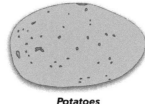
Potatoes

Phosphorus

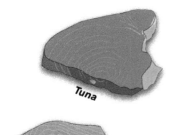
Tuna

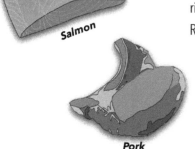
Salmon

Phosphorus is needed to produce ATP (the energy molecule), regulating bone and teeth strength, proper cell functioning, and regulating body pH levels. Deficiencies in Phosphorus can lead to Rickets, weakened immune system, anaemia, muscle pain, decreased appetite, and numbness. Excess Phosphorus is quite serious and causes more Calcium to be released from bone stores into the bloodstream, which can lead to calcification (i.e. hardening) of the internal organs and blood vessels. This can dramatically increase the risk for cardiovascular diseases such as heart attacks and strokes[27]. The RDA for Phosphorus is **700 mg/day (men & women)**.

Pork

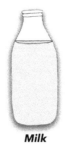
Milk

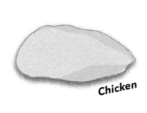
Chicken

Sulfur

Sulfur is the third most abundant mineral within your body and is obtained in the diet from protein almost exclusively. As a result, sulfur does not currently have an RDA. Sulfur is an intermediary component of key metabolites such as glutathione and therefore is needed to maintain nitrogen balance. Protein sulfur deficiency may result in protein-energy malnutrition[28].

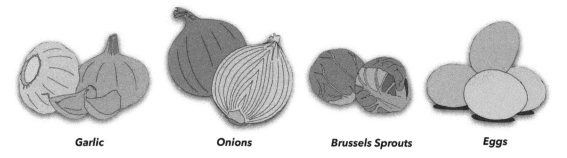

| **Garlic** | **Onions** | **Brussels Sprouts** | **Eggs** |

Trace Minerals

Chromium

Chromium enhances the effects of insulin, the hormone responsible for the regulation of blood sugar levels and the metabolism of carbohydrates, fats, and lipids in the body[29]. Chromium is found in two forms: *trivalent* (Chromium 3+), which is the biologically active form that's found in food, and *hexavalent* (Chromium 6+), which is a toxic form that comes from industrial pollution. Deficiencies in Chromium are rare, however, low levels may lead to blood glucose control issues that may increase the risk for developing type 2 diabetes. There are no known issues with excess Chromium intake and as such there are no calculated tolerable upper limits. Chromium is found in a wide range of foods but is low in simple sugars. Supplemental use of Brewer's Yeast has traditionally been recommended for improving blood glucose control due to its high concentration of Chromium. Brewer's Yeast can be used by all populations but is most beneficial to those with diabetes[30]. The RDA for Chromium is **35 µg/day (men)** and **25 µg/day (women)**. These values decrease at 50 years old to 30 µg/day and 20 µg/day respectively.

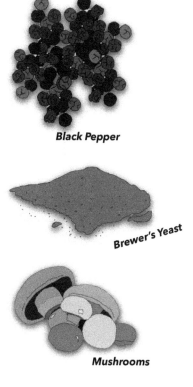

Black Pepper

Brewer's Yeast

Mushrooms

Copper

Copper is found in all bodily tissues with the highest concentration present in the liver, brain, heart, kidneys, and skeletal muscles. Copper is a cofactor for several enzymes called *cuproenzymes*, which aid in red blood cell production, maintaining nerve signalling, energy production, collagen formation, and iron absorption. Copper also has physiological roles including neurohormone homeostasis, regulating gene expression, healthy brain development, and immune system function[31]. Deficiencies in copper whilst rare have been linked to cardiovascular disease and nervous system dysfunction. Excess copper levels are more common and may lead to Menke's, Wilson's, and Alzheimer's disease. The RDA from Copper is **900 µg/day (men & women)**.

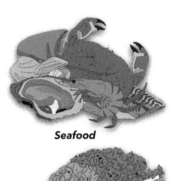

Seafood

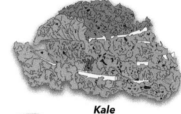

Kale

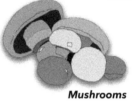

Mushrooms

Sesame Seeds

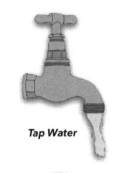

Tap Water

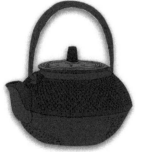

Tea

Fluoride

Fluoride is present in the body as calcium fluoride and forms part of healthy bones and teeth. Fluoride is most well known for its benefits in preventing tooth decay and is usually added to tap water through a process called fluoridation. Seawater is a source of sodium fluoride. Food prepared using tap water and seafood all contain good amounts of fluoride as well as tea[32]. Excess fluoride is very rare and usually only shows in infants consuming fluoride only from baby formula. The RDA for Fluoride is **4 mg/day (men)**, or **3 mg/day (women)**.

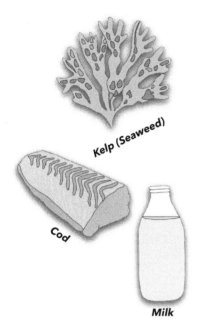

Kelp (Seaweed)

Cod

Milk

Iodine

Iodine is an essential component of the thyroid hormones *triiodothyronine (t3)* and *thyroxine (t4)*. Thyroid hormones regulate several biochemical reactions within the body including protein synthesis and are a key factor in healthy metabolic activity. Iodine may also have physiological roles in immune function. Iodine is best found in kelp, cod, and milk but can also be obtained from crops grown in iodine-rich soil[33]. Iodine deficiencies are rare but may lead to thyroid-related health complications and may affect growth and development in infants. Excess iodine can cause thyroid inflammation called a *goitre* and thyroid cancer. The RDA for Iodine is **150 µg/day (men & women)**.

Iron

Iron is a key component of several molecules within the body. For example, *Haem* (Iron-containing compound) is found in Haemoglobin and Myoglobin, which transport oxygen in the red blood cells and muscles repetitively[34]. Therefore, if the oxygen-carrying capacity is reduced due to low Iron levels, then aerobic performance/endurance may also be impaired. Dietary iron comes in two forms: *Haem Iron* and *Non-Haem Iron*. Plant sources of iron only contain non-haem iron, whereas meat, seafood, and poultry contain both haem iron and non-haem iron. Haem iron is more bioavailable than non-haem iron, as well as being less affected by other dietary nutrients (see Chapter 4). Iron deficiency (a.k.a. *anaemia*) is not uncommon in women of reproductive age and vegetarians/vegans[35]. Iron deficiency symptoms may include low energy levels, gastrointestinal issues, weakness, and problems with memory and concentration. Excess iron may also cause complications such as constipation, nausea, abdominal pain, fainting, convulsions, coma, and even death[36]. The RDA for iron is **8 mg/day (men)** or **18 mg/day (women)**. Iron level requirements for women may decrease once reaching the menopause to 8 mg/day.

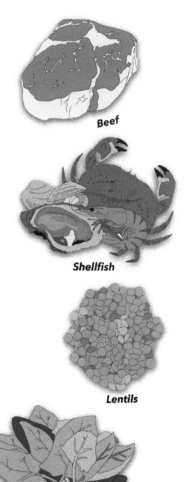

Beef

Shellfish

Lentils

Spinach

Manganese

Manganese acts as a cofactor to several key enzymes (e.g. *Superoxide Dismutase*, *Arginase*, and *Pyruvate Carboxylase*), that are involved in the metabolism of amino acids, cholesterol, glucose, and carbohydrates; scavenging of reactive oxygen species (ROS); aid in bone formation; assist in reproduction; and support your immune response. Manganese also assists Vitamin K in maintaining *haemostasis* (haemostasis = the regulation of blood flow) through blood clotting[37]. Most of the manganese within your body is found in your bones with the remainder concentrated within the liver, pancreas, kidneys, and brain. Manganese deficiency and toxicity from excess manganese is rare, outside of industrial workers such as welders and miners. However, some evidence suggests that low manganese may be linked to poor bone quality and retarded growth. Excess manganese may cause symptoms of tremors, muscle spasms, hearing loss, tinnitus, and loss of balance. The RDA for Manganese is **2.3 mg/day (men)** or **1.8 mg/day (women)**.

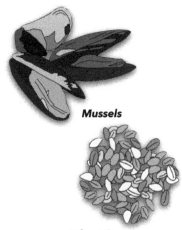
Mussels

Wheat Germ

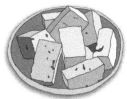
Tofu

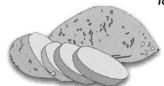
Sweet Potato

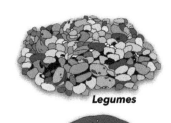
Legumes

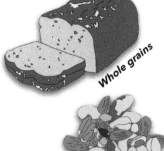
Whole grains

Molybdenum

Molybdenum is a structural component of a cofactor called *Molybdopterin* that is needed for the function of the enzymes *Sulfite Oxidase*, *Xanthine Oxidase*, *Aldehyde Oxidase*, and *Mitochondrial Amidoxime Reducing Component (mARC)*. These enzymes are involved in metabolising drugs, toxins, sulfur-containing amino acids, and heterocyclic compounds such as purines and pyrimidines[38]. Molybdenum deficiency is only seen in rare genetic mutation cases but can cause seizures and neurological damage. Excess molybdenum levels are also rare but can occur in industrial workers causing gout-like symptoms. The RDA for Molybdenum is **45 µg/day (men & women)**.

Nuts

Selenium

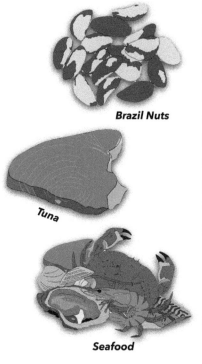

Brazil Nuts

Tuna

Selenium is found as inorganic (*Selenate* and *Selenite*) and organic selenium (*Selenomethionine* and *Selenocysteine*) and is needed in thyroid hormone metabolism, DNA synthesis, reproduction, and protection from oxidative damage and infection[39]. Selenium deficiency alone may not cause ill health but may predispose you to other illness when experienced in combination with other stresses. For example, selenium deficiency in combination with a viral infection may cause Keshan disease. Excess selenium may present as a strong garlic odour breath or metallic taste can cause nail/hair loss, rashes, nausea, diarrhoea, fatigue, and irritability. The RDA for Selenium is **55 µg/day (men & women)**.

Seafood

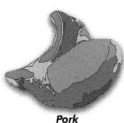

Pork

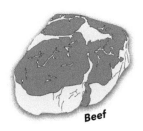

Beef

Zinc

More than 100 different enzymes are zinc-dependent. Zinc is needed for the structure of cell membranes and some proteins, acts as a stabiliser for other proteins, decreases vulnerability to oxidative damage, and plays a role in cell signalling including hormonal control, nerve conduction, and programmed cell death[40]. Zinc deficiency can lead to a decreased sense of smell/taste, poor wound healing, unexplained weight loss, lack of alertness, loss of appetite, open skin sores, dry skin conditions, weakened immune system, diarrhoea, poor cognitive function and learning ability, and possible mental health conditions such as Schizophrenia. The RDA for Zinc is **11 mg/day (men)** or **8 mg/day (women)**.

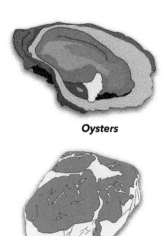

Oysters

Beef

Vitamins (units)	RDA/AI (Men)	RDA/AI (Women)	Maximum	Best Non-Fortified Sources
Vitamin A (µg/day)	900	700	3,000	Sweet Potato, Carrots, Tuna, Butternut Squash
Thiamine (B1) (mg/day)	1.2	1.1	Unknown	Pork, Salmon, Flaxseed
Riboflavin (B2) (mg/day)	1.3	1.1	Unknown	Beef, Milk, Salmon, Mushrooms
Niacin (B3) (mg/day)	16	14	35	Tuna, Chicken, Pork, Beef
Pantothenic Acid (B5) (mg/day)	5	5	Unknown	Mushrooms, Salmon, Avocados
Vitamin B6 (mg/d)	1.3	1.3	100	Salmon, Chicken, Pork, Beef
Biotin (B7) (µg/d)	30	30	Unknown	Liver, Kidneys, Egg Yolks, Nuts
Folate (B9) (µg/d)	400	400	1,000	Lentils, Asparagus, Spinach
Vitamin B12 (µg/d)	2.4	2.4	Unknown	Clams, Liver, Mackerel, Crab
Vitamin C (mg/day)	90	75	2,000	Guavas, Peppers, Kiwifruit
Vitamin D (µg/day)	15	15	100	Sunlight (UVB), Salmon
Vitamin E (mg/day)	15	15	1,000	Sunflower Seeds, Almonds
Vitamin K (µg/day)	120	90	Unknown	Kale, Broccoli, Brussels Sprouts, Cabbage

Disclaimer: All the above recommended daily allowances are for healthy adults aged 18 - 70 years old and an average TDEE of 2,000 calories/day.[41] Recommendations may be different for very active adults, adolescents, pregnant or lactating women or those with diagnosed deficiencies or diseases. The above guidelines do not replace the advice of a medical professional and you should always consult your doctor if you have any concerns about your health or potential deficiencies.

Minerals (units)	RDA/AI (Men)	RDA/AI (Women)	Maximum	Best Non-Fortified Sources
Calcium (mg/day)	1,000	1,000	2,500	Milk, Yoghurt, Cheese
Chloride (g/day)	2.3	2.3	3.6	Salt, Kelp (Seaweed), Tomatoes, Lettuce, Olives
Chromium (µg/day)	35	25	Unknown	Black Pepper, Brewer's Yeast, Mushrooms
Copper (µg/day)	900	900	10,000	Seafood, Kale, Mushrooms, Sesame Seeds
Fluoride (mg/day)	4	3	10	Tea, Tap Water
Iodine (µg/day)	150	150	1,100	Kelp (seaweed), Cod, Milk
Iron (mg/day)	8	18	45	Beef, Shellfish, Lentils, Kidney Beans, Spinach
Magnesium (mg/day)	400	310	350	Spinach, Seeds, Beans
Manganese (mg/day)	2.3	1.8	11	Mussels, Wheat Germ, Tofu, Sweet Potatoes
Molybdenum (µg/day)	45	45	2,000	Legumes, Wholegrains, Nuts
Phosphorus (mg/day)	700	700	4,000	Tuna, Salmon, Pork, Milk, Chicken
Potassium (g/day)	4.7	4.7	Unknown	Salmon, Lima Beans, Avocados, Potatoes, Bananas
Selenium (µg/day)	55	55	400	Brazil Nuts, Tuna, Seafood, Pork, Beef
Sodium (g/day)	1.5	1.5	2.3	Salt
Sulfur	n/a	n/a	Unknown	Garlic, Onions, Brussel Sprouts, Eggs
Zinc (mg/day)	11	8	40	Oysters, Beef

Disclaimer: All the above recommended daily allowances are for healthy adults aged 18 - 70 years old and an average TDEE of 2,000 calories/day.[42] Recommendations may be different for very active adults, adolescents, pregnant or lactating women or those with diagnosed deficiencies or diseases. The above guidelines do not replace the advice of a medical professional and you should always consult your doctor if you have any concerns about your health or potential deficiencies.

Hydration

Staying adequately hydrated is possibly one of the most undervalued things you can do to improve your health and performance. Good hydration improves kidney function, helps keep your skin well moisturised, improves alertness and concentration, improves digestion, helps regulate healthy blood pressure, prevents early fatiguing, improves thermoregulation (i.e. body temperature control), prevents poor endurance and more[43]. Water comprises around 45 - 70% of total body mass and is largely dependent upon total fat mass, with an average weight man containing around 35 - 55 litres of total body water. Fat has a relatively low water content of approx. 10 - 15% of its total mass, whereas lean tissue (e.g. muscle mass), has a water content of approx. 75% of its total mass. Therefore, the more body fat you have, the less water you will have in your body. However, it is important to understand that total body water content is not a measurement of hydration, nor should it be used as a guide for fluid intake.

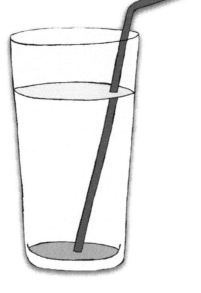

Water is found in the body in two places: within each cell (*Intracellular Fluid*) or outside of the cells (*Extracellular Fluid*). The water within the body is not plain water, as it contains several

Electrolytes (substances that produce an electrical conducting solution when dissolved in water). Electrolytes are either positively charged *Cations* (e.g. Sodium, Potassium, Calcium, and Magnesium), or negatively charged *Anions* (e.g. Chloride and Bicarbonate). The concentration of these electrolytes is not constant throughout the body and will differ depending on the location within the body and the local needs[44]. Electrolytes help to keep the body in a state of water balance known as *Euhydration*. Euhydration in its simplest definition is where there is an adequate amount of water within the body, no more, no less. When there is negative water balance within the body (insufficient water content) this is known as *Hypohydration*, whereas a positive water balance within the body (excess water content) is known as *Hyperhydration*.

Trying to achieve Euhydration is a constant process, where you will fluctuate between states of dehydration (losing body water) and rehydration (gaining body water). However, total body water will only vary by around 0.5%. Despite this relatively small fluctuation to total body water, dehydration can have a significant effect on your health and performance.

For example, dehydration can lead to urinary and kidney problems such as urinary tract infections (UTIs), kidney stones, and kidney failure; seizures due to electrolyte imbalances; hypovolemic shock (low oxygen to organs due to low blood volume), impaired mental state and confusion, dry skin conditions such as eczema, and more[45]. The effects of dehydration can vary in severity based upon the percentage you are dehydrated as shown below.

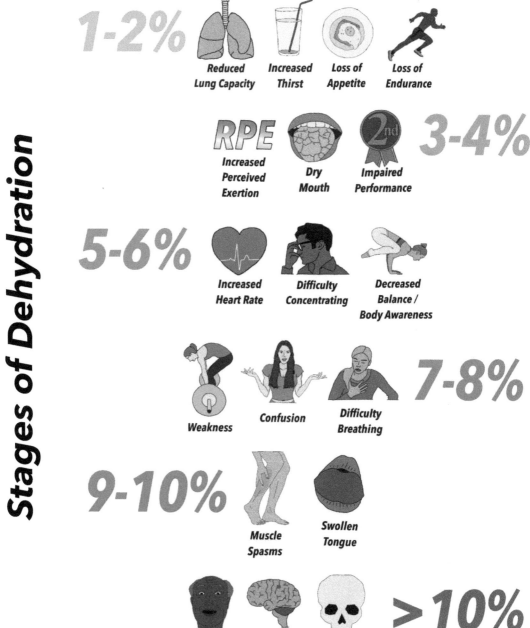

Practical Applications

You should always adopt a food first approach to getting all your essential macro- and micronutrients. A multivitamin supplement can be used in addition to a healthy, well-balanced, and diverse diet as a sort of "insurance policy" but should never be used as a substitute for a good diet. The clue is in the name - **supplements should "supplement" a good diet not replace it**. However, you may need to use vitamin/mineral supplementation if you are at higher risk of deficiency (i.e. Vitamin B12 and Iron deficiency for vegetarians/vegans; vitamin D deficiency between October to April for those living in the Northern Hemisphere; or if you have been advised to take supplements by a qualified medical professional).

Micronutrient Colour Guide

The easiest way to ensure adequate amounts of each vitamin and mineral are achieved from your diet is to first include as much variety and diversity as possible to your diet. An easy way to do this is by focusing on eating as many different colours of fruits, vegetables, nuts, seeds, fish, meat, dairy, eggs, grains, pulses, and legumes. Many key vitamins and minerals tend to be found together in different coloured foods including key *Phytonutrients* that aid in the absorption of vitamins and minerals. Chemicals within your food that aid in the absorption of key nutrients are called bioenhancers and will be covered in Chapter 5 - Bioavailability.

Orange/Yellow Foods

Foods that are orange/yellow are often high in carotenoids and are a great source of fibre and Vitamin A. Orange/yellow foods are generally seen as beneficial for skin and eye health, improve immune function, decrease your risk of cancer and heart disease, and help to keep joints healthy[46]. One tip to increase non-heam iron absorption is to drink citrus juices (e.g. orange juice) with plant iron sources (e.g. spinach, lentils).

Red Foods

Red coloured fruit and vegetables contain phytonutrients including lycopene and anthocyanins, which is where they get their vibrant red colour. These phytonutrients boost the effects of other key vitamins and minerals and are associated with reducing cancer, diabetes, and type 2 diabetes risk, improving skin quality, and lowering the risk of macular degeneration (an age-related eye condition)[46]. One key tip for enhancing the effects of lycopene (particularly in tomatoes) is to consume them cooked in soups, stews, or even with olive oil and some seasoning.

Blue /Purple Foods

Blue and purple foods are high in resveratrol and anthocyanin. These phytonutrients give them their unique colour and provide anti-ageing and anti-inflammatory properties. Blue and purple foods also reduce your risk of Alzheimer's disease, improves cognitive function and memory, and reduces cancer risk[46]. Although red wine is often celebrated for its health benefits, it is the resveratrol within it that provides these benefits. Therefore, if you choose not to drink alcohol you can still get the benefits by eating grapes and berries instead. If you do drink alcohol, ensure you stay within the healthy limits of < 14 units/week.

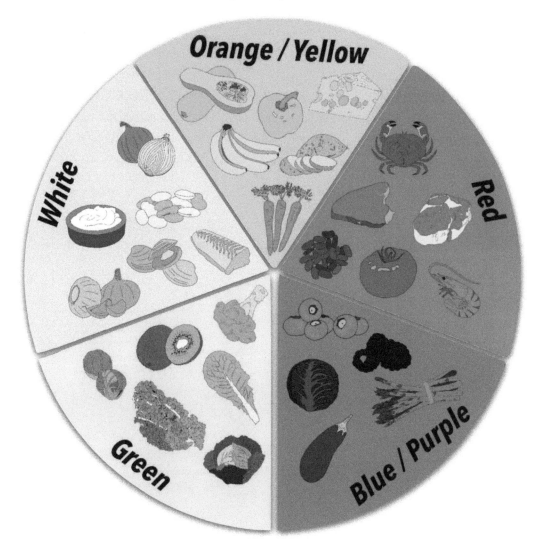

Green Foods

Green foods get their colour from chlorophyll (which is what plants use to generate energy from the sun). Green foods are packed with anti-oxidants that aid in healing, digestion, and immunity, as well as reducing your risk of cancer and are a good source of fibre[46]. A tip for people wanting to reduce their carbohydrate intake is to use courgette (a.k.a. zucchini) to make "spaghetti" with the aid of a spiralizer.

White Foods

Technically, white isn't a colour, however, white foods do possess several health benefits as they contain the phytonutrients anthoxanthins, allicin, and quercetin. White colour foods garlic, onions, potatoes, cauliflower etc. can help protect against cancer, maintain bone strength, lower heart disease risk, reduce inflammation and provide prebiotics for your gut microbiome[46]. A tip for cooking potatoes is to let them cool before serving which lowers their glycemic index and increases resistant starch levels.

Hydration Strategies

Government recommendations for water (or fluid) intake across the world are developed to provide a single number that fits a large majority of the population, based upon average age and weight. As a result, the most commonly quoted recommendations for water intake are 1.5 L/day (women) and 2.0 L/day (men). However, this generic number may be inadequate for a large proportion of the population who are not average age or weight. Various National Dietetics Associations have provided more detailed recommendations for fluid intake and I have detailed the information you need to calculate your hydration needs below[47]:

Age	Recommended Fluid Intake (ml/kg of bodyweight/day)
16 - 30	35 - 40
31 - 54	30 - 35
55 - 65	30
Over 65	25

As an example:

at 41 years old and 93 kg, Mr Couch-Potato should have between 2.79 and 3.26 L/day.
(i.e. 30 ml x 93 kg = 2,790 ml, 2,790 ml / 1,000 = 2.79 L/day)

Now you know how much fluid you need to drink each day you need to consider how you're going to get all this fluid effectively. Firstly, fluid intake includes all liquids that you drink, not just water. In fact, while water is a good default option for fluid intake there are other drinks which hydrate just as well and some even better than water[48]. However, I would advise against anyone using juices and soft drinks as their main source of fluid intake. Fluid intake also includes the water found in the food you eat. Approximately, 500ml of your fluid intake may be achieved through your food alone, however, this is dependent upon the foods you eat. For example, fruit and vegetables are around 90 - 95% water, whereas processed meats like bacon are only around 12% water (see table opposite)[49]. *A simplified strategy to ensure you are staying well-hydrated is to have 400-500 ml of water with each of your 3 main meals and sip from a water bottle between meals.*

Sources	% Water Content
Water	100
Milk, Strawberries, Watermelon, Lettuce, Cabbage, Celery, Spinach, Pickles.	90 - 99
Fruit Juice, Yoghurt, Apples, Grapes, Oranges, Carrots, Broccoli (cooked), Pineapple	80 - 89
Bananas, Avocados, Cottage Cheese, Ricotta Cheese, Potato (baked), Shrimp	70 - 79
Pasta (cooked), Legumes, Salmon, Ice Cream, Chicken Breast	60 - 69
Ground Beef, Hotdogs, Feta Cheese, Tenderloin Steak (cooked)	50 - 59
Pizza	40 - 49
Cheddar Cheese, Bagels, Bread	30 - 39
Pepperoni Sausage, Cakes, Biscuits	20 - 29
Butter, Margarine, Raisins, Bacon	10 - 19
Nuts, Pretzels, Peanut Butter, Crackers	1 - 9
Oils, Sugars	0

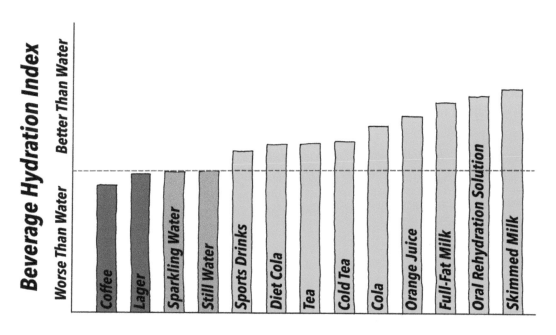

Graph adapted from Maughan et al (2015).

Monitoring Hydration Status

Much like TDEE calculations, it is important to understand that water requirement calculations are an estimate of your needs and it is prudent to have an objective way to try to assess if you are staying adequately hydrated. The gold standard for monitoring hydration status is urine osmolality. However, cheaper and more assessable methods such as urine specific gravity (dip-stick test), urine colour, or bodyweight fluctuations pre- and post-workouts may be preferred.

Plasma Osmolality

Osmolality is a measurement of the concentration of particles within the fluid. *When in a state of euhydration, plasma osmolality is maintained around a set point of approx. 285 mOsm/kg*[50]. Plasma volume decreases when sweating which increases the concentration of particles within the plasma and the osmolality score. *Plasma osmolality increases by approx. 5 mOsm/kg for every 2% loss in bodyweight from sweating*[51]. While this gold standard of measuring hydration status is useful for medics and sport scientists, it may not be very practical for the average person. Therefore, the methods below may provide a suitable alternative.

Body Weight

As most of the weight lost during a single exercise bout will be water, any lost weight can be converted into fluid intake needs. 1 kg is equivalent to 214 ml of fluid. Therefore, *for every 1 kg difference between pre- and post-exercise weight, aim to consume 214 ml of fluid in addition to your calculated daily intake*[52]. For example, as Ms Gym-Bunny weighs 55 kg before exercise and 53.6 kg post-exercise she should consume an additional 300 ml of fluid to adequately rehydrate. If you are hydrating during your workouts you may notice no significant change in your weight and this is a crude indication of a good hydration strategy.

Specific Gravity

Specific gravity is a measurement of the concentration of your urine, relative to water. *A urine specific gravity reading of less than 1.010 indicates that you are chronically well-hydrated*. Readings between 1.011 and 1.020 indicate mild chronic dehydration, 1.021 – 1.030 indicates significant chronic dehydration, and readings above 1.030 indicate serious chronic dehydration and an immediate need to rehydrate[53].

Urine Colour Guide

The colour of your urine is possibly the most well-known self-guide on checking your hydration levels, with a *pale straw/yellow urine colour indicating good levels of hydration*. However, your urine colour is a crude guide to hydration status and may be affected by other factors (e.g. supplements, diet, and disease). Urine colour also only gives an acute (short-term) look at your hydration levels[54]. Despite these limitations, this is one of the easiest hydration checks available and when used in combination with the above calculations for hydration needs, it can be a useful tool. Therefore, below is a guide to different urine colours and what this means to your hydration strategy.

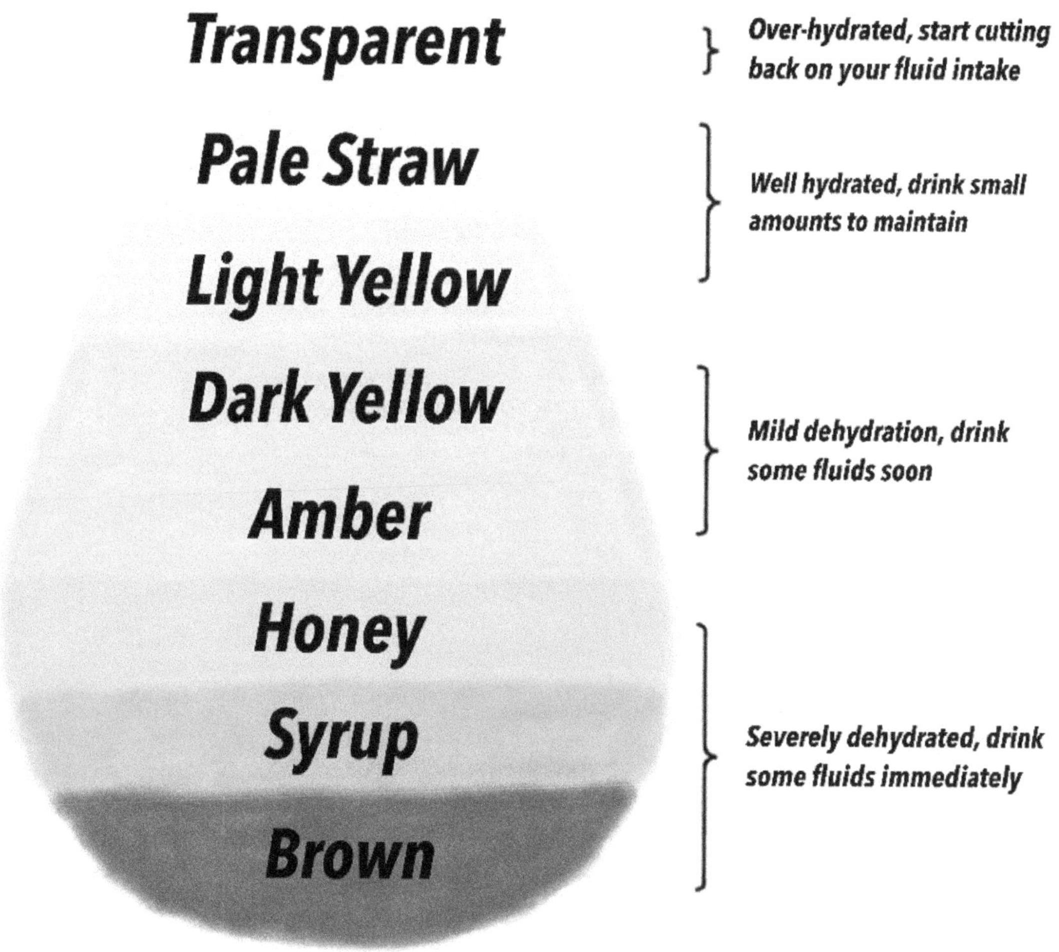

Transparent } *Over-hydrated, start cutting back on your fluid intake*

Pale Straw

Light Yellow *Well hydrated, drink small amounts to maintain*

Dark Yellow

Amber *Mild dehydration, drink some fluids soon*

Honey

Syrup

Brown *Severely dehydrated, drink some fluids immediately*

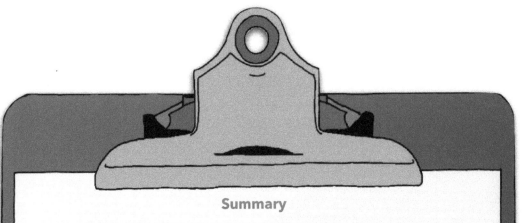

Summary

✓ Micronutrients consist of Vitamins and Minerals. There are **13 Vitamins** which are either water-soluble or fat-soluble depending on how they travel within your body. There are **16 minerals** which are considered either macrominerals or trace elements based on how much is needed in your diet.

✓ **Vitamins and minerals are defined by whether insufficient amounts are detrimental to health and the restoration of said vitamin/mineral will prevent or cure symptoms**.

✓ Water-soluble vitamin include **Vitamin C** and the **B Vitamins (B1, B2, B3, B5, B6, B7, B9, B12)**. Fat-soluble vitamins include **Vitamin A, D, E, and K**.

✓ Macrominerals include **Calcium, Chloride, Magnesium, Sodium, Potassium, Phosphorus, and Sulfur**. Trace minerals include **Chromium, Copper, Fluoride, Iodine, Iron, Manganese, Molybdenum, Selenium, and Zinc.**

✓ **The human body is 45 - 70% water and is directly related to body fat mass**.

✓ Body water is stored within cells (**intracellular fluid**) or outside of the cells (**extracellular water**).

✓ The water within your body contains **Electrolytes** that help to maintain water balance through varying concentrations of **Cations** and **Anions**.

✓ Water balance is also called **Euhydration** where there is adequate water no more, no less. You will fluctuate between periods of negative water balance (**Hypohydration**) and periods of positive water balance (**Hyperhydration**). When you are losing water to regain water balance you are dehydrating and when gaining water you are rehydrating.

✓ The easiest way to get sufficient micronutrients from your diet is to **include a lot of diversity including foods from each of the 5 main colours**: Orange/Yellow, Red, Blue/Purple, Green, and White.

✓ Your water needs are primarily determined by your age, weight, and activity levels.

✓ **All fluid hydrates you including the fluid found in your food**. While water should be your default fluid of choice, **some fluids may hydrate better or worse than water**.

✓ The foods with the highest water content are fruits, vegetables, and gains that absorb water during cooking (e.g. pasta, rice, etc.).

✓ You can monitor your hydration status using **Plasma Osmolality, Body Weight, Specific Gravity, or Urine Colour**.

✓ When using urine colour as a guide to hydration a pale colour but not transparent is the ideal.

REFERENCES

[1] Antonio, J. et al. (2008), *Essentials of Sports Nutrition and Supplements*, Humana Press

[2] Gibney, M. J., Lanham-New, S. A., Cassidy, A., and Vorster, H. H., (2009), *Introduction to Human Nutrition*, Wiley-Blackwell

[3] Patient. (2020), *Hypervitaminosis*, Retrieved from https://patient.info/doctor/hypervitaminosis

[4] National Institutes of Health, (2020), *Thiamin: Fact Sheet for Health Professionals*, Retrieved from https://ods.od.nih.gov/factsheets/Thiamin-HealthProfessional/

[5] National Institutes of Health, (2020), *Riboflavin: Fact Sheet for Health Professionals*, Retrieved from https://ods.od.nih.gov/factsheets/Riboflavin-HealthProfessional/

[6] National Institutes of Health, (2020), *Niacin: Fact Sheet for Health Professionals*, Retrieved from https://ods.od.nih.gov/factsheets/Niacin-HealthProfessional/

[7] National Institutes of Health, (2020), *Pantothenic Acid: Fact Sheet for Health Professionals*, Retrieved from https://ods.od.nih.gov/factsheets/PantothenicAcid-HealthProfessional/

[8] National Institutes of Health, (2020), *Vitamin B6: Fact Sheet for Health Professionals*, Retrieved from https://ods.od.nih.gov/factsheets/VitaminB6-HealthProfessional/

[9] National Institutes of Health, (2020), *Biotin: Fact Sheet for Health Professionals*, Retrieved from https://ods.od.nih.gov/factsheets/Biotin-HealthProfessional/

[10] National Institutes of Health, (2020), *Folate: Fact Sheet for Health Professionals*, Retrieved from https://ods.od.nih.gov/factsheets/Folate-HealthProfessional/

[11] National Institutes of Health, (2020), *Vitamin B12: Fact Sheet for Health Professionals*, Retrieved from https://ods.od.nih.gov/factsheets/VitaminB12-HealthProfessional/

[12] National Institutes of Health, (2020), *Vitamin C: Fact Sheet for Health Professional*, Retrieved from https://ods.od.nih.gov/factsheets/VitaminC-HealthProfessional/

[13] Baron, J. H., (2009), *Sailors' scurvy before and after James Lind - a reassessment*, Nutrition Reviews, 67(6), 315-332 https://doi.org/10.1111/j.1753-4887.2009.00205.x

[14] National Institutes of Health, (2020), *Vitamin A: Fact Sheet for Health Professionals*, Retrieved from https://ods.od.nih.gov/factsheets/VitaminA-HealthProfessional/

[15] National Institutes of Health, (2020), *Vitamin D: Fact Sheet for Health Professionals*, Retrieved from https://ods.od.nih.gov/factsheets/VitaminD-HealthProfessional/

[16] National Institutes of Health, (2020), *Vitamin E: Fact Sheet for Health Professionals*, Retrieved from https://ods.od.nih.gov/factsheets/VitaminE-HealthProfessional/

[17] National Institutes of Health, (2020), *Vitamin K: Fact Sheet for Health Professionals*, Retrieved from https://ods.od.nih.gov/factsheets/vitaminK-HealthProfessional/

[18] Karl, J. P., Meydani, M. Barnett, et al., (2017), *Fecal concentrations of bacterially derived vitamin K forms are associated with gut microbiota composition but not plasma or fecal cytokine concentrations in healthy adults*, American Journal of Clinical Nutrition. 106(4), 1052-1061. https://doi.org/10.3945/ajcn.117.155424

[19] Hyman, M., (2011), *Eat Your Medicine: Food As Pharmacology*, Retrieved from https://www.huffpost.com/entry/food-as-medicine_b_1011805

[20] National Institutes of Health, (2020), *Calcium: Fact Sheet for Health Professionals*, Retrieved from https://ods.od.nih.gov/factsheets/Calcium-HealthProfessional/

[21] Tortora, G. J. & Derrickson, B., (2017), *Principles of Anatomy & Physiology*, Wiley & Sons Inc.

[22] MedlinePlus, (2020), *Chloride in diet*, Retrieved from https://medlineplus.gov/ency/article/002417.htm

[23] National Institutes of Health, (2020), *Magnesium: Fact Sheet for Health Professionals*, Retrieved from https://ods.od.nih.gov/factsheets/Magnesium-HealthProfessional/

[24] MedlinePlus, (2020), *Sodium in diet*, Retrieved from https://medlineplus.gov/ency/article/002415.htm

[25] Valentine V. (2007), *The importance of salt in the athlete's diet*. Current Sports Medicine Reports, 6(4), 237-240, https://doi.org/10.1007/s11932-007-0038-3

[26] National Institutes of Health, (2020), *Potassium: Fact Sheet for Health Professionals*, Retrieved from https://ods.od.nih.gov/factsheets/Potassium-HealthProfessional/

[27] National Institutes of Health, (2020), *Phosphorus: Fact Sheet for Health Professionals*, Retrieved from https://ods.od.nih.gov/factsheets/Phosphorus-HealthProfessional/

[28] Nimni, M. E., Han, B., and Cordoba, F., (2007), *Are we getting enough sulfur in our diet?*, Nutrition & Metabolism, 4, 24, https://doi.org/10.1186/1743-7075-4-24

[29] National Institutes of Health, (2020), *Chromium: Fact Sheet for Health Professionals*, Retrieved from https://ods.od.nih.gov/factsheets/Chromium-HealthProfessional/

[30] Hosseinzadeh, P., Javanbakht, M. H., Mostafavi, S. A., Djalali, M., Derakhshanian, H., Hajianfar, H., ... Djazayer, A. (2013). *Brewer's yeast improves glycemic indices in type 2 diabetes mellitus*. International Journal of Preventive Medicine, 4(10), 1131-1138,

[31] National Institutes of Health, (2020), *Copper: Fact Sheet for Health Professionals*, Retrieved from https://ods.od.nih.gov/factsheets/Copper-HealthProfessional/

[32] MedlinePlus, (2020), *Fluoride in diet*, Retrieved from https://medlineplus.gov/ency/article/002420.htm

[33] National Institutes of Health, (2020), *Iodine: Fact Sheet for Health Professionals*, Retrieved from https://ods.od.nih.gov/factsheets/Iodine-HealthProfessional/

[34] National Institutes of Health, (2020), *Iron: Fact Sheet for Health Professionals*, Retrieved from https://ods.od.nih.gov/factsheets/Iron-HealthProfessional/

[35] Saunders, A. V., Craig, W. J., Baines, S. K., and Posen, J. S., (2013), *Iron and vegetarian diets*, Medical Journal of Australia, 199 (4), S11-S16, https://doi.org/10.5694/mja11.11494

[36] National Institutes of Health, (2020), *Iron: Fact Sheet for Health Professionals*, Retrieved from https://ods.od.nih.gov/factsheets/Iron-HealthProfessional/

[37] National Institutes of Health, (2020), *Manganese: Fact Sheet for Health Professionals*, Retrieved from https://ods.od.nih.gov/factsheets/Manganese-HealthProfessional/

38 National Institutes of Health, (2020), *Molybdenum: Fact Sheet for Health Professionals*, Retrieved from https://ods.od.nih.gov/factsheets/Molybdenum-HealthProfessional/

39 National Institutes of Health, (2020), *Selenium: Fact Sheet for Health Professionals*, Retrieved from https://ods.od.nih.gov/factsheets/Selenium-HealthProfessional/

40 National Institutes of Health, (2020), *Zinc: Fact Sheet for Health Professionals*, Retrieved from https://ods.od.nih.gov/factsheets/Zinc-HealthProfessional/

41 Institute of Medicine, Food and Nutrition Board, (2011), *Dietary Reference Intakes (DRIs): Recommended Dietary Allowances and Adequate Intakes, Vitamins*, Retrieved from https://www.ncbi.nlm.nih.gov/books/NBK56068/table/summarytables.t2/?report=objectonly

42 Institute of Medicine, Food and Nutrition Board, (2011), *Dietary Reference Intakes (DRIs): Recommended Dietary Allowances and Adequate Intakes, Elements*, Retrieved from https://www.ncbi.nlm.nih.gov/books/NBK545442/table/appJ_tab3/?report=objectonly

43 Popkin, B. M., D'Anci, K. E., and Rosenberg, I. H., (2010), *Water, Hydration and Health*, Nutrition Reviews, 68(8), 439-458, https://ww.ncbi.nlm.nih.gov/pmc/articles/PMC2908954/

44 Campbell, C. I., & Spano, M. A., (2011), *NSCA's Guide to Sport and Exercise Nutrition*, Human Kinetics

45 Mayo Clinic, (2020), *Dehydration*, Retrieved from https://www.mayoclinic.org/diseases-conditions/dehydration/symptoms-causes/syc-20354086

46 Minich, D. N., (2019), *A Review of the Science of Colorful, Plant-Based Food and Practical Strategies for "Eating the Rainbow"*, Journal of Nutrition and Metabolism, Article ID 2125070, https://doi.org/10.1155/2019/2125070

47 Vivanti, A. P., (2012), *Origins for the estimations of water requirements in adults*, European Journal of Clinical Nutrition, 66, 1282-1289, https://www.nature.com/articles/ejcn2012157

48 Maughan, R., J., Watson, P., Cordery, P. A. et al., (2015), *A Randomized Trial to Assessthe Potential of Different Beverages to Affect Hydration Status: Development of a Beverage Hydration Index*, American Journal of Clinical Nutrition, 103 (3), 717-723, https://doi.org/10.3945/ajcn.115.114769

49 Popkin, B. M., D'Anci, K. E., and Rosenberg, I. H., (2010), *Water, Hydration and Health*, Nutrition Reviews, 68(8), 439-458, https://www.ncbi.nlm.nih.gov/pmc/articles/PMC2908954/

50 Panel on Dietary Reference Intakes for Electrolytes and Water. Chapter 4, Water, In: *Dietary Reference Intakes for Water, Potassium, Sodium, Chloride, and Sulfate*. Washington, D.C.: Institute of Medicine, National Academy Press, pp. 73-185, 2005.

51 Popowski, L.A., R.A. Oppliger, G.P. Lambert, R.F. Johnson, A.K. Johnson, and C.V. Gisolfi (2001). *Blood and urinary measures of hydration during progressive acute dehydration*. Medical Science of Sports Exercise, 33, 747-753

52 Campbell, C. I., & Spano, M. A., (2011), *NSCA's Guide to Sport and Exercise Nutrition*, Human Kinetics

53 University of Utah Medical School, (2020), *Urinalysis*, Retrieved from https://webpath.med.utah.edu/TUTORIAL/URINE/URINE.html

54 NHS, (2020), *Hydration*, Retrieved from https://www.nhsinform.scot/campaigns/hydration

4

MEAL FREQUENCY & TIMING

How many meals a day and when should I eat them?

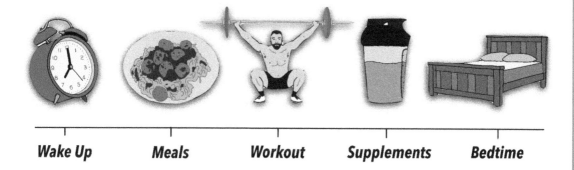

| **Wake Up** | **Meals** | **Workout** | **Supplements** | **Bedtime** |

We calculated in the previous chapters how many calories you need to consume and how much of this should come from each macronutrient to achieve your goals. While knowing how much/what to eat is extremely important, you may also want to know when and how often to eat specific foods to maximise your potential and reach your goals. The timing and frequency of your meals need to be personalised to you and your needs, not only to achieve your goals but also to make your diet sustainable and enjoyable. Nutrient timing can be defined as *"the consumption of nutrients in and around an exercise bout to optimise muscular adaptation and/or performance"*.[1] Meal Frequency put simply is *how many meals/snacks you consume per day*. While there has been a good amount of research into the timing of nutrient intake there has been significantly less research conducted into meal frequency, particularly in athletic populations. Despite limitations in the available research, a detailed guide on how you can implement meal frequency and timing strategies into your nutrition plan is provided based on the evidence available and some practical experience too.

Eating Non-Stop or All In One Go

A very common debate in the health and fitness community is whether it is better to eat larger meals less often or to eat frequent smaller meals when trying to improve your health and aid in weight loss. Despite this common debate, there are limited amounts of quality research examining the physiological effects of meal frequency on human health. However, there is some evidence to refute some common diet myths around meal frequency.

Weight Loss and Health Markers

Most of us know someone who has achieved great improvements to their health and lost excess weight by using diet strategies that seem to focus purely on meal frequency. For example, some people swear by eating just one large meal per day whereas others say snacking between meals helps with their hunger cravings so they don't overeat at mealtimes. However, *the benefits of meal frequency-based diets are derived from being more mindful of what you are eating and reducing your total caloric intake*. This is why either end of the spectrum of meals per day can produce similar results[2]. Being more mindful of what you are eating will often translate to an increase in fibre and nutrient-dense foods, and a reduction in processed and convenience foods. These actions in combination with a reduction in excess weight are all positively correlated with improvements in cholesterol, blood glucose control, and blood pressure.

Boosting Your Metabolism & Reducing Hunger

A commonly proposed benefit of increased meal frequency is increasing your metabolism by either raising your basal metabolic rate (BMR) or increasing the thermic effect of food (TEF). Although research in this area has only involved short duration studies, several reviews of gold-standard studies conducted in metabolic chambers has shown *there is no significant difference in basal metabolic rate or thermic effect of food when comparing anywhere between one and six meals per day*.[3,4] Therefore, the number of meals you choose to consume per day should not be dictated by ideas of "stoking the metabolic fire" and should be based on personal preference and tolerance. Eating more frequently has also been suggested as a way to decrease appetite and hunger cravings. However, research to date shows the effects of meal frequency on appetite and hunger have focused solely on same-day hunger levels and more long-term research in this area is absent. While eating smaller snacks before main meals have been shown to decrease total calories consumed, it does not affect perceived hunger levels[5]. A more useful tactic may be to focus on consuming more satiating foods such as protein and fibre, which have been shown to reduce both perceived hunger levels and the total number of calories consumed[6,7].

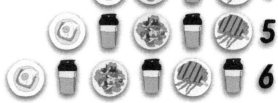

Retaining Lean Muscle Mass

It has been well established that muscle protein synthesis (MPS) is optimised with a 20 - 30g dose of protein (or 10 - 15g of essential amino acids), so you'd be forgiven for thinking the more times you can stimulate MPS per day the more lean mass you can build or retain. While some research has shown a positive benefit from increased meal frequency and greater lean mass retention[8], these studies have flawed methodology and the protein intake between groups was not equal. In fact, *research on meal frequency and changes in body composition have found no significant difference in lean mass retention between eating 3 or 6 meals per day*.[9] Ultimately, it is more important to focus on reaching your daily protein requirements rather than how many times you are eating protein per day.

Timing is Everything, or is it?

The International Society of Sports Nutrition (ISSN) defines nutrient timing as *"the purposeful ingestion of all types of nutrients at various times throughout the day to favourably impact the adaptive response to acute and chronic exercise"*.[10] However, the timing of your meals has also received a lot of attention on its potential benefits on general health. In obese and sedentary individuals there is some

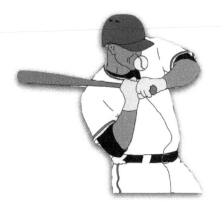

evidence to suggest eating the majority of your calories in the morning may produce greater amounts of weight loss, when compared to eating the majority of your daily calories in the evening[11,12]. A notable caveat to this research was the morning eaters also lost more lean muscle mass and as such this may be detrimental to long-term weight maintenance. Other limitations include diet adherence was assessed by self-reporting with is known to suffer from a large amount of under-reporting; there was no exercise component to either study, and there is a lack of comparison to an even meal distribution pattern. As a result, these results cannot be translated to the general population, particularly those who are more physically active. *For general health, the timing of your meals should be dictated by what you can adhere to and help you stay within your caloric needs*. When it comes to enhancing the adaptive response to exercise or your performance there are benefits to strategically planning your macronutrient intake. The benefits of micronutrient timing are predominately on increasing nutrient bioavailability and as such will be covered separately in Chapter 5.

The Anabolic Window - Fact or Fiction?

If you've ever spent a significant length of time in a gym then you may have heard about the anabolic window or heard statements such as "I don't want to lose my gains" followed by some gym-bro downing their protein shake a mere seconds after finishing their last set. But what is the anabolic window and is there any truth to its existence? The source of this 'broscience' is research conducted in Denmark on older men who saw a loss of strength and lean muscle mass when not consuming protein within 2-hours post-workout[13]. Over time the advertised length of the anabolic window has become shorter and shorter as many gym-bros and supplement companies have repeated this piece of info and now some claim you need to eat protein within 20 minutes of

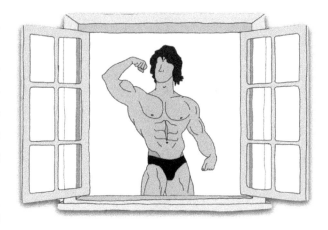

finishing your last set or you'll lose your gains completely. Without getting too bogged down in the science this doesn't make sense from a physiological standpoint and the anabolic window as described above is pure fiction.

Exercise itself is catabolic (**catabolic** = tissue breakdown) but, exercise also increases the sensitivity of your muscles to amino acid uptake, which is the first step into moving into an anabolic state (**anabolic** = tissue building). However, your muscles will not move into an anabolic state unless they receive adequate dietary protein to create a positive nitrogen balance. Your muscles are sensitised to MPS for between 24 and 72-hours following an acute bout of exercise. Beginner lifters will experience longer increases in sensitivity than experienced lifters who are closer to their genetic muscular potential. Research comparing eating protein before or after a bout of exercise has shown no significant differences in muscular hypertrophy or strength gains. Also, while the research does show a benefit to consuming protein within a 4 hours window (2 hours before to 2 hours after) a bout of exercise, the effect of this on overall improvements in muscular size and strength are minimal if you are consuming your ideal daily amount of protein[14]. The take-home message here is *if possible, try to consume protein within a 4-hour window of exercise but if you can't or don't want to, then you'll still make progress if you're meeting your daily protein requirements*.

What is Carbohydrate Loading and Fat Loading?

As discussed in the previous chapters your body has a limited ability to store carbohydrates and once your glycogen stores are depleted you return to burning fat as your default source of fuel. A drawback of this is the intensity of exercise you can complete is reduced due to the slower ATP production from slow glycolysis and the oxidative system. By understanding this process it becomes clear the benefit of maximising your body's stores of glycogen to ensure you can compete at higher intensities for as long as possible. *Glycogen stores are maximised by following a high-carbohydrate diet of 8 - 12 g/kg/day*.[15] By eating a high amount of excess calories as carbohydrates you have a sufficient surplus to load more glycogen into your stores, which is where the phrase "carb-loading" comes from. If you are completing a one-off endurance event with plenty of time to prepare, eating a high-carbohydrate diet in the days preceding your event is enough to maximise your glycogen stores. The issue of timing is more critical when you are performing extended/multiple bouts of endurance-based exercise or if you have limited recovery time before you need to perform again. Increased carbohydrate intake can also benefit resistance-based exercise to maximise muscle glycogen stores, improve muscle damage, and improve acute and chronic adaptation to resistance training.

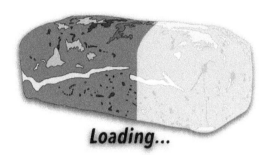

Loading...

Fat loading is a newer concept which focuses on trying to enhance your metabolic efficiency by alternating between periods of high-carb, low-fat and high-fat, low-carb to help "train" your body to utilise fat stores for longer during exercise before switching to using glycogen stores. This practice can theoretically help you work harder for longer and potentially improve your performance. For more information on fat loading see the metabolic efficiency section of Chapter 2.

Practical Applications

General Health & Well-being

If your focus is to remain in good health, manage a healthy weight, and reduce your risk of disease, then meal timing and frequency plays a much less significant role than it does for those looking to gain a performance advantage. However, the number of meals you have per day may help you to adhere to your chosen diet format. For example, if you are not hungry in the morning and prefer to eat 2 large meals per day then this may be a good option for you. If you find yourself wanting to snack during the day then planning to have smaller main meals to accommodate more frequent eating, then this option may work for you instead. *Whatever amount of meals you feel you can stick with and stay on track to reach your goals is the right amount for you*. There is no one size fits all.

Protein Frequency & Timing

The number of times per day you eat protein and the timing of your protein intake should be dictated by your daily protein intake requirements to reach your goals and potentially trying to capitalise on opportunities to stimulate muscle protein synthesis (although this is far less significant than total daily protein intake). As previously mentioned, *MPS is maximised with doses of 20 - 30 g of protein per meal* and doses above this threshold show no significant increase in muscle protein synthesis. This does not mean that any protein above this amount per meal will be wasted, rather protein intake above this threshold will be used to repair other tissues in the body instead. Therefore, the number of meals/snacks you eat per day will be determined by how many times you hit this threshold per day and your personal preferences. This could mean that someone may eat just one meal/day within the 4-hour window of training or at the other end of the spectrum, someone else may eat 6 meals/day including breakfast, lunch, dinner, snacks before and after training and a pre-bedtime feeding. While a number of meals/day can work well, a general guide of 3 - 6 meals/day is the most practical and well-tolerated by most. An alternate way to maximise muscle protein synthesis and calculate your protein requirements per meal is to *aim for a target of 0.25 - 0.40 grams/kilogram/meal and trying to eat every 4 hours*.[16] To help explain how you can implement these strategies we'll use Mr Hard-Gainer and his goal to gain more lean muscle mass.

- Mr Hard-Gainer's daily protein requirements are 1.6 - 2.2 g/kg/day which is equivalent to 96 - 132 g of protein. For our calculations, we'll use a **target of 120 g/day** (equal to 2.0 g/kg/day).
- As the optimum amount of protein to stimulate MPS is **20 - 30 g per meal** this would mean Mr Hard-Gainer needs to eat **4 - 6 meals/day** with 20 - 30 grams of protein to optimise his protein intake (**120 / 30 = 4 meals/day, 120 / 20 = 6 meals/day**).
- Alternatively, using the 0.25 - 0.40 g/kg/meal guide, Mr Hard-Gainer could aim for **15 - 24 grams of protein every 4 hours** (around 4 - 5 meals/day).
- Capitalising on the 4-hour anabolic window around exercise and nighttime feeding this could include breakfast, lunch, and dinner, with a high protein snack before training, quick-release whey protein after exercise and slow release casein protein before bed.

Nighttime Feeding

With each feeding opportunity, there is a spike in MPS, however, overnight this decreases significantly and this time has been identified as a missed opportunity to stimulate MPS. Research has shown that *drinking a slow releasing protein (e.g. casein) beverage 30 minutes before bedtime increases MPS, enhances recovery, and has no negative effects on health*[17,18]. To optimise this opportunity the research suggests 30 - 40 grams of casein protein 30 minutes before bedtime, however, capitalising on any individual opportunity to stimulate muscle protein synthesis should always come second to meeting your daily protein requirements.

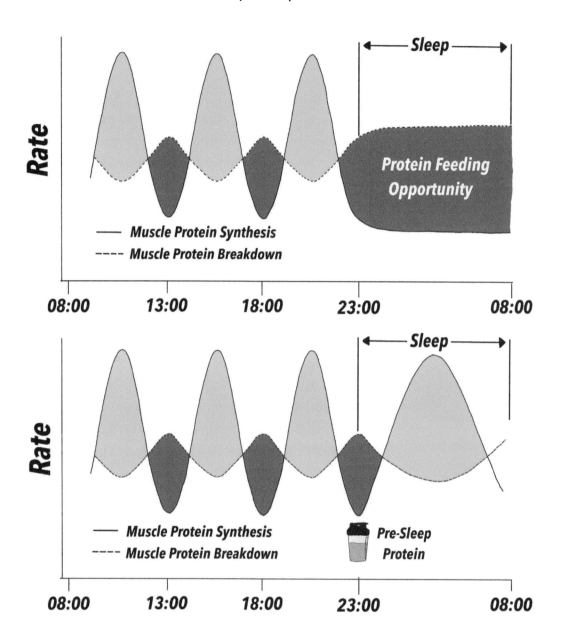

Carbohydrate Frequency & Timing

Prolonged (> 60 - 90 minutes) moderate- to high-intensity exercise is heavily reliant upon your glycogen stores[19] and therefore strategically altering your carbohydrate intake to increase glycogen stores can have a significant effect on your performance and is one of the most well-studied techniques in all of sports nutrition. Depending on what type of exercise you are engaged in and the length of time you plan to exercise, you may want to increase your carbohydrate intake to ensure you have enough "fuel" to stay performing at your best.

To keep things as clear as possible this section is divided into strategies to support endurance-based exercise and resistance-based exercise.

Endurance-based Exercise

Increasing your carbohydrate intake in the days preceding an endurance-based event will maximise your glycogen stores and improve your performance on the day. This strategy is even more important for those following a low-carbohydrate diet as their glycogen stores may be significantly depleted and will be unable to perform at their best without a carb-loading strategy. A good strategy to follow is to *ingest a high-carbohydrate diet of 8 - 12 g/kg/day while simultaneously reducing your training volume for the 1 - 3 days leading up to your endurance-based event*.[20] Men and women have different levels of carbohydrate/fat utilisation[21]. Therefore, women may need to increase caloric intake and eat on the higher end of this carb-loading range to achieve similar effects to men.

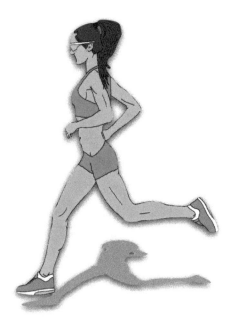

During any prolonged endurance event, you may also benefit from trying to *attenuate glycogen depletion by ingesting simple carbohydrates during your event such as 30 - 60 g of carbohydrates in 150 - 350 ml of electrolyte fluid solution every 10 - 15 minutes*. Alternatively, a 5-second oral rinse of the same solution but spitting out the solution may also provide similar results, but the mechanisms behind this are not yet fully understood[22]. Following an endurance-based event returning to a normal eating pattern will see the replenishment of your glycogen stores to base levels within a few days. However, if you are engaged in more regular endurance-based events (e.g. team sports athletes playing multiple times per day or multi-event competitions), then you may not have 3 - 4 days to optimise your glycogen stores through a traditional loading strategy. In these circumstances where you need *to rapidly replenish your glycogen stores, you should consume 1.2 g/kg/hour with a preference for high-glycemic carbohydrates (GI > 70) for 4 - 6 hours after exhausting exercise*. You may also benefit from eating a combination of both glucose and fructose sugars, adding 3 - 8 mg/kg of caffeine, and 0.2 - 0.5 g/kg/hour of protein to aid glycogen re-synthesis. For ultra-endurance events lasting greater than 8 hours, the same 8 - 12 g/kg/day carbohydrate loading strategy is still sufficient, however, the importance of restoring your glucose levels during competition are increased.

Carbohydrate & Protein Requirements Before, During, and After Endurance Events

	No Time Restraints	<4h Recovery Time
Before	High-carb diet (8 - 12 g/kg/day) for 1 - 3 days leading up to event. Goal to maintain glycogen levels in hour before event (1 - 4 g/kg) of carbs.	High-carb diet (8 - 12 g/kg/day) for 1 - 3 days leading up to event. Goal to maintain glycogen levels in hour before event (1 - 4 g/kg) of carbs.
During	30 - 60 g of carbs in 150 - 350 ml of electrolyte solution every 10 - 15 minutes or oral rinse.	30 - 60 g of carbs in 150 - 350 ml of electrolyte solution every 10 - 15 minutes or oral rinse.
After	Return to normal macronutrient distribution and eating behaviours.	1.2 g/kg/hour of carbs 3 - 8 mg/kg of caffeine 0.2 - 0.5g/kg/hour of protein

Notes: You should always try to meet the bulk of your caloric needs through a varied food first approach. Any food timing and frequency strategies should also be tested first in training to ensure they are well tolerated and does not impede your performance on game day.

Resistance-based Exercise

During resistance-based exercise, glycogen levels decline significantly limiting your ability to maintain exercise intensity[23] and increasing the rate of tissue breakdown[24]. As both of these factors may limit the amount of strength and muscular hypertrophy you can achieve, it is prudent to ensure you are eating enough carbohydrates to support your workouts and goals. The goal here should be to eat enough carbohydrates per day to maximise your glycogen stores, based on the volume and intensity of exercise you plan to complete (see Chapter 2). While the research into the benefits of timing your carbohydrate intake for resistance-based exercise is limited, or with mixed results, there has been some research to suggest there may be some benefits of *consuming carbohydrates alone or in combination with protein pre- and post-exercise to help increase glycogen stores, improve muscle damage, and facilitate greater training adaptations*[25,26]. When meeting your daily carbohydrate intake goals you may want to include a larger amount of your carbohydrates pre- and post-exercise, but only if this does not cause you any digestive distress (e.g. bloating, cramps, gas), which may impede your performance. The size of your pre-exercise meal may reduce the amount you need to eat in your post-exercise meal and still achieve an ergogenic benefit (**ergogenic** = enhances physical performance). Therefore, *if you consume a high-carb, high-protein meal before your workout you may only need a smaller amount of carbs in your post-workout meal*.

Hydration for Performance

If you are engaged in extended bouts of exercise or competitive events you may need more structure to your hydration strategy than detailed in Chapter 3, to ensure you do not see any decreases in your performance[27]. The recommendation for how much fluid you should consume can be divided into three time periods: before, during, and after exercise.

Before Exercise

- Goal is to start exercise in a state of euhydration.
- Slowly *drink approx. 5 - 7 ml/kg of bodyweight at least 4h before exercise*. If no urine produced or dark in colour drink approx. 3 - 5 ml/kg of bodyweight more until pale in colour or until urine output returns to normal.
- Consuming *beverages with 20 - 50 mEq/L (**mEq/L** = milliequivalent per litre) of sodium, eating salty snacks, or higher sodium foods may aid in retaining more fluids and stimulate thirst*.
- There is no significant benefit to trying to hyper-hydrate before exercise and this may increase your need to void your bladder during exercise.

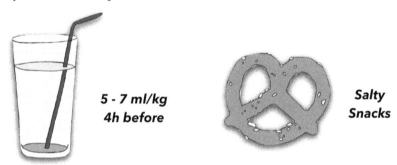

5 - 7 ml/kg
4h before

Salty
Snacks

During Exercise

- Goal is to prevent excessive dehydration of greater than 2% of bodyweight from water losses and excessive changes in electrolyte balance that may hinder performance.
- Aim to drink periodically during exercise where exercise task permits (i.e. using water station or during time-outs).
- Fluid replacement needs are determined by sweat loss, exercise duration and number of hydration opportunities.
- Sweat rates vary greatly, however, *drinking between 0.4 - 0.8 litres/hour is a good general guide*. Athletes with heavier sweat rates; are heavier in weight, or exercising in hotter environments should aim for the higher end of this range, whereas lighter weight, lighter sweaters, or cold environment exercisers should aim for the lower end of the range.

- Monitoring your bodyweight pre- and post-workouts is the most accurate way to understand what amount of fluid you need to consume to reach euhydration during exercise. This will ensure that come event day you are properly prepared.
- The consumption of beverages containing electrolytes and carbohydrates can also help sustain fluid balance and exercise performance. *Beverages with approx. 20 - 30 mEq/L of sodium, approx. 2 - 5 mEq/L of potassium, and approx. 5 - 10% or 30 - 60 g/hour of carbohydrates is optimum for maintaining hydration status during extended bouts of exercise (i.e. >1 h).*

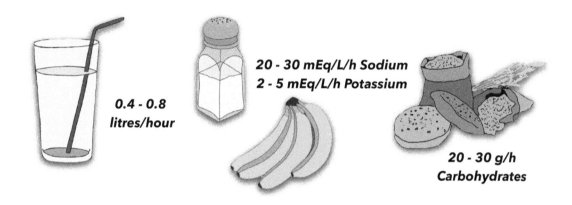

0.4 - 0.8 litres/hour

**20 - 30 mEq/L/h Sodium
2 - 5 mEq/L/h Potassium**

**20 - 30 g/h
Carbohydrates**

After Exercise

- Goal is to fully replace the fluid and electrolytes lost during exercise.
- How aggressive your rehydration strategy needs to be is based upon when you next need to compete/exercise again.
- If time permits, returning to normal hydration and food intake will bring you back to euhydration.
- *If dehydration is substantial or your recovery time is short (i.e. <12 hours), then a more aggressive strategy of approx. 1.5 litres of electrolyte-containing fluids per kilogram of bodyweight lost* is recommended and spread out as much as possible to help with fluid retention.

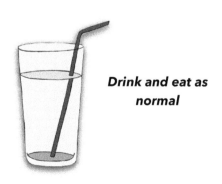

**Drink and eat as
normal**

Planned Re-feeds

When you are eating within a calorie deficit it can be more difficult to retain lean muscle mass. It can also be quite mentally draining eating fewer and fewer calories each week to keep making progress. This is where including strategically timed re-feeds can be particularly beneficial. A re-feed is a day where you deliberately increase your caloric intake to aid diet adherence and maintain lean muscle mass[28]. The simplest way to include re-feeds is when planning your daily caloric deficit. For example, we know that a 500 calorie/day deficit equals 3,500 calories/week (equivalent to 1 pound of body fat). However, as long as your weekly calorie deficit remains the same then each day does not need to be in a calorie deficit and the amount can vary quite a bit. To help explain we'll use Mr Couch-Potato from Chapter 1 and his weight loss goals.

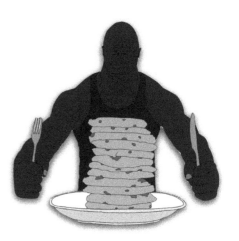

- Mr Couch-Potato has a TDEE of 2,284 calories/day and a **calorie deficit goal of 3,900 calories/week**.
- To achieve his goal Mr Couch-Potato can either evenly divide 3,900 calories across the week (557 calories/day deficit), or he can divide it unevenly to allow for planned re-feeds.
- For example, Mr Couch-Potato is prone to eating more on weekends and wants to plan for this. Therefore, Mr Couch-Potato decides to have a **780 calorie/day deficit Monday to Friday** and then **eats his TDEE on Saturday & Sunday** to still reach his target weight loss.
- Therefore, Mr Couch Potato would have a **target caloric intake of 1,504 calories/day on weekdays and 2,284 calories/day on weekends**.

An uneven daily calorie restriction can help create the feeling of not dieting every day, as some days you will be able to eat considerably more than others and can allow for occasional treats or special events. However, these 're-feed' days are not an excuse to binge and eat as much as you like in a more typical 'cheat day' format.

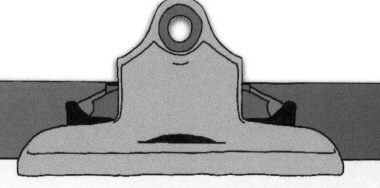

Summary

✓ **Meal frequency does not have a significant effect on improving your body composition.**

✓ **Meal frequency does not significantly affect your total daily energy expenditure, the thermic effect of food, or your resting metabolic rate.**

✓ Evidence to support increasing or decreasing meal frequency on improving health markers (e.g. cholesterol, blood glucose, insulin etc.) is mixed at best and **your chosen meal frequency may be determined solely by personal preference and tolerance**.

✓ **There is no significant evidence to support increasing meal frequency will help in reducing your hunger levels**.

✓ If protein intake is optimised at each feeding opportunity and across the day, **the number of meals per day may have no significant impact on performance and lean muscle mass retention.**

✓ **The Anabolic Window is much larger than many would think and last from approx. 2 hours before to 2 hours after about of resistance-based exercise**. However, meeting your total daily protein requirements has a greater effect on muscle protein synthesis (MPS) as opposed to focusing on eating within the anabolic window.

✓ **Carb-Loading is an effective way to increase your glycogen stores to help increase work capacity** during both endurance-based and resistance-based exercise.

✓ Eating slow-releasing protein (e.g. Casein) before bedtime can help increase MPS during the natural low that occurs during nighttime fasting without any adverse health effects.

✓ Uneven caloric restrictions to include **Re-Feeds are an effective tool to help with diet adherence and to increase lean muscle mass retention during extended periods of caloric restriction**.

REFERENCES

1 Aragon, A. A., & Schoenfeld, B. J., (2013), *Nutrient timing revisited: is there a post-exercise anabolic window?*. Journal of the International Society of Sports Nutrition, 10(1), 5, https://doi.org/10.1186/1550-2783-10-5

2 Schoenfeld, B. J., Aragon, A. A., and Krueger, J.W., (2015), *Effects of meal frequency on weight loss and body composition: a meta-analysis*. Nutrition Reviews, 73(2), 69 - 82 https://doi.org/10.1093/nutrit/nuu017

3 Calcagno, M., Kahleova, H., Alwarith, J., Burgess, N. N., Flores, R. A., Busta, M. L., & Barnard, N. D., (2019), *The Thermic Effect of Food: A Review*, Journal of the American College of Nutrition, 38:6, 547-551, https://doi.org/10.1080/07315724.2018.1552544

4 La Bounty, P. M., Campbell, B. I., Wilson, J., Galvan, E., Berardi, J., Kleiner, S. M., Kreider, R. B., Stout, J. R., Ziegenfuss, T., Spano, M., Smith, A., and Antonio, J., (2011), *International Society of Sports Nutrition position stand: meal frequency*, Journal of the International Society of Sports Nutrition, 8(4), https://doi.org/10.1186/1550-2783-8-4

5 Leidy, H. J. & Campbell, W. W., (2011), *The effect of eating frequency on appetite control and food intake: brief synopsis of controlled feeding studies*. The Journal of Nutrition, 141(1), 154 - 7 https://doi.org/10.3945/jn.109.114389

6 Paddon-Jones, D., Westman, E., Mattes, R. D., Wolfe, R. R., Astrup, A., and Westerterp-Plantenga, M., (2008), *Protein, weight management, and satiety*, The American Journal of Clinical Nutrition, 87(5), 1558S–1561S, https://doi.org/10.1093/ajcn/87.5.1558S

7 Slavin, J. and Green, H. (2007), *Dietary fibre and satiety*. Nutrition Bulletin, 32: 32-42. https://doi.org/10.1111/j.1467-3010.2007.00603.x

8 Iwao, S., Mori, K. and Sato, Y. (1996), *Effects of meal frequency on body composition during weight control in boxers*. Scandinavian Journal of Medicine & Science in Sports, 6: 265-272. https://doi.org/10.1111/j.1600-0838.1996.tb00469.x

9 Cameron, J., Cyr, M., & Doucet, É. (2010). *Increased meal frequency does not promote greater weight loss in subjects who were prescribed an 8-week equi-energetic energy-restricted diet.* British Journal of Nutrition, 103(8), 1098-1101. https://doi.org/10.1017/S0007114509992984

10 Kerksick, C. M., Arent, S., Schoenfeld, B. J., Stout, J. R., Campbell, B., Wilborn, C. D., Taylor, L., Kalman, D., Smith-Ryan, A. E., Kreider, R. B., Willoughby, D., Arciero, P. J., VanDusseldrop, T. A., Ormsbee, M. J., Wildman, R., Greenwood, M., Ziegenfuss, T. N., Aragon, A. A., and Antonio, J., (2007), *International society of sports nutrition position stand: nutrient timing*. Journal of the International Society of Sports Nutrition, 14, 33, https://doi.org/10.1186/s12970-017-0189-4

11 Jakubowicz D, Barnea M, Wainstein J, Froy O., (2013), *High Caloric Intake At Breakfast Vs. Dinner Differentially Influences Weight Loss Of Overweight And Obese Women*. Obesity; 21(12): 2504–12. https://doi.org/10.1002/oby.20460

12 Ma Y, Bertone ER, Stanek EJ 3rd, Reed GW, Hebert JR, Cohen NL, Merriam PA, Ockene IS., (2003), *Association Between Eating Patterns And Obesity In A FreeLiving Us Adult Population*. American Journal of Epidemiology. 158(1): 85–92. https://doi.org/10.1093/aje/kwg117

13 Esmarck, B., Andersen, J. L., Olsen, S., Richter, E. A., Mizuno, M.,and Kjaer, M., (2001), *Timing of postexercise protein intake is important for muscle hypertrophy with resistance training in elderly humans*. Journal of Physiology. 535(Pt 1), 301-311, https://doi.org/10.1111/j.1469-7793.2001.00301.x

14 Aragon, A.A., Schoenfeld, B.J. (2013). *Nutrient timing revisited: is there a post-exercise anabolic window?*. Journal of the International Society of Sports Nutrition, 10, 5. https://doi.org/10.1186/1550-2783-10-5

15 Karlsson, J.,and Saltin, B., (1971), *Diet, Muscle Glycogen, And Endurance Performance*. Journal of Applied Physiology. 31(2):203–6.

16 Schoenfeld, B.J., Aragon, A.A., (2018), *How much protein can the body use in a single meal for muscle-building? Implications for daily protein distribution*. *Journal of the International Society of Sports Nutrition, 15*, 10. https://doi.org/10.1186/s12970-018-0215-1

17 Res P., Groen, B., Pennings, B., Beelen, M., Wallis, G. A., Gijsen, A. P., Senden, J. M., Vanl, L. J., (2012), *Protein Ingestion Before Sleep Improves Postexercise Overnight Recovery*. Medical Science of Sports Exercise, 44(8), 1560–9.

18 Groen, B. B., Res, P. T., Pennings, B., Hertle, E., Senden, J. M., Saris, W. H., Van Loon, L. J., (2012), *Intragastric Protein Administration Stimulates Overnight Muscle Protein Synthesis In Elderly Men*. American Journal of Physiology Endocrinology Metabolism. 302(1), E52–60.

19 Kerksick, C. M., Arent, S., Schoenfeld, B. J., Stout, J. R., Campbell, B., Wilborn, C. D., Taylor, L., Kalman, D., Smith-Ryan, A. E., Kreider, R. B., Willoughby, D., Arciero, P. J., VanDusseldrop, T. A., Ormsbee, M. J., Wildman, R., Greenwood, M., Ziegenfuss, T. N., Aragon, A. A., and Antonio, J., (2007), *International society of sports nutrition position stand: nutrient timing*. Journal of the International Society of Sports Nutrition, 14, 33, https://doi.org/10.1186/s12970-017-0189-4

20 Fairchild, T. J., Fletcher, S., Steele, P., Goodman, C., Dawson, B., Fournier, P. A., (2002), *Rapid Carbohydrate Loading After A Short Bout Of Near Maximal-Intensity Exercise*. Medicine and Science of Sports Exercise. 34(6):980–6.

21 Wismann, J., and Willoughby, D., (2006), *Gender Differences In Carbohydrate Metabolism And Carbohydrate Loading*. Journal of the International Society of Sports Nutrition. 3:28–34.

22 Jeukendrup, A. E., (2013), *Oral Carbohydrate Rinse: Placebo or Beneficial?*, Current Sports Medicine Reports: 12 (4), 222-227, https://doi.org/10.1249/JSR.0b013e31829a6caa

23 Coyle EF, Coggan AR, Hemmert MK, Lowe RC, Walters TJ., (1985), *Substrate Usage During Prolonged Exercise Following A Preexercise Meal*. Journal of Applied Physiology, 59(2), 429–433.

24 Rodriguez, N. R., Di Marco, N. M., Langley, S., (2009), *American College Of Sports Medicine Position Stand*. Nutrition And Athletic Performance. Medicine and Science in Sports Exercise, 41(3), 709–731.

25 Tipton, K. D., Rasmussen, B. B., Miller, S. L., Wolf, S.E., Owens-Stovall, S. K., Petrini, B. E., Wolfe, R. R., (2001), *Timing Of Amino Acid-Carbohydrate Ingestion Alters Anabolic Response Of Muscle To Resistance Exercise*. American Journal of Physiology and Endocrinology Metabolism, 281(2):E197–206.

26 White, J. P., Wilson, J. M., Austin, K. G., Greer, B. K., St John, N., Panton, L. B., (2008), *Effect Of Carbohydrate-Protein Supplement Timing On Acute Exercise-Induced Muscle Damage.* Journal of the International Society of Sports Nutrition. 5:5.

27 Campbell, C. I., & Spano, M. A., (2011), *NSCA's Guide to Sport and Exercise Nutrition*, Human Kinetics

28 Campbell et al. (2020). *Intermittent Energy Restriction Attenuates the Loss of Fat Free Mass in Resistance Trained Individuals. A Randomized Controlled Trial.* Journal of Functional Morphology and Kinesiology, 5(1), 19; https://doi.org/10.3390/jfmk5010019

5

BIOAVAILABILITY

How much of what you eat can you digest and use?

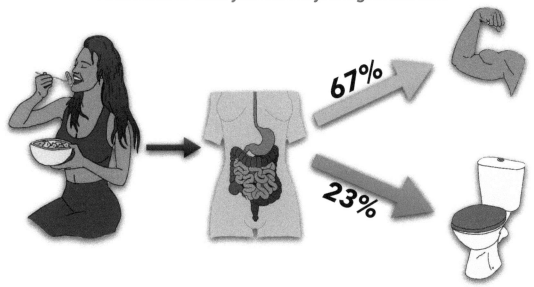

Every time you consume food or drink, the nutrients contained within the food/drink source are released from the matrix and absorbed into the bloodstream, where they are transported to wherever they are needed for normal bodily functions. However, not all the nutrients in your food and drink can be utilised to the same extent. This is known as *Bioavailability* and it can have a significant effect on your health and performance.

Bioavailability Explained

From ingestion to excretion, the food you consume may encounter several factors that affect your body's ability to utilise the macro- and micronutrients effectively. These include internal factors such as gender, age, pregnancy, and nutritional status (e.g. being malnourished), as well as external factors such as the chemical form of the ingested nutrients and nutrients consumed within the same meal/day[1]. Both macronutrients (mostly protein) and micronutrients are affected by these factors and it is important to understand bioavailability to ensure you can optimise your nutrition for promoting good health and high-level performance.

The first step in making a given nutrient bioavailable is to liberate the nutrients from the food matrix and turn it into a chemical form that can bind and enter the cells or pass between them. This process is known as **bioaccessibility** and is achieved by chewing (**mastication**), initial digestion in the mouth by key enzymes, mixing the food with the stomach acid, and the release of the foods into the small intestine, where the food receives more enzymes via the pancreas and where the majority of digestion occurs[2]. Cooking significantly helps with the digestibility of food, particularly plant foods. For example, raw vegetables are a great source of many different nutrients, however, cooking some plant foods helps their nutrients to be released from the matrix more freely, increasing the amount that you can extract and utilise[3]. The reason cooking your food is so beneficial stems back to when humans evolved millions of years ago from eating a plant-only diet and our intestines reduced in length, due to a reduced amount of time needed to absorb nutrients from your food[4]. This information is often overlooked by more extreme diet practices such as raw-food veganism and can lead to nutrient deficiencies.

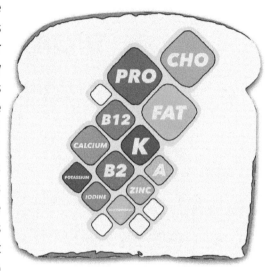

Different nutrients can interact with each other and may have either an inhibitory, enhancing, or no effect on nutrient bioavailability, if enhancer and inhibitor effects are equal. Enhancers can work in many different ways including maintaining the solubility of the nutrients or by protecting it from interaction with inhibitors. Inhibitors may reduce nutrient bioavailability by binding a nutrient into a form not recognised by the cells, making the nutrient insoluble, and/or competing for the same nutrient uptake system[5]. An example of competing nutrients for the same uptake system is calcium and non-haem iron, which both bind to the surface of intestinal absorptive cells. This can be thought of as the calcium standing in a doorway and stopping the non-haem iron from getting through.

Key vitamins and minerals are often added to foods to increase their nutritional value through a process called **fortification**. A good example of this is where some key nutrients are added to cereals and flours to help increase their presence in the diet[6]. This does not mean you should only consume fortified foods, rather some fortified foods may help ensure you meet your minimum recommended daily allowance (RDA) when eaten in combination with natural dietary sources. Your age, gender, and health status also affect nutrient bioavailability. For example, if you are deficient in one nutrient due to a change in your physiological state (e.g. pregnancy), then your body will adapt by increasing the absorptive pathways for that nutrient. Absorptive pathways for calcium and zinc are examples of nutrients regulated in this manner. However, some medical conditions, particularly *inflammatory conditions or infections may reduce your gut's absorptive* *ability*, for example, low iron absorption when suffering from a common cold. Other examples of host factors on bioavailability include decreased B12 absorption as you age and low iron levels during menstruation.

Protein Quality

Protein quality refers to *"the ability of a specific dietary protein to support body growth and maintenance"*. There have been many different methods used to determine protein quality over the years with 2 key assessment methods still in widespread use. These are the *Protein Digestibility Corrected Amino Acid Score (PDCAAS)* and the *Digestibility Indispensable Amino Acid Score (DIAAS)*. The DIAAS is the newer of these methods and is now the gold standard in assessing protein quality. However, as the test is still relatively new there is not a complete body of data for all isolated protein and mixed protein sources so the PDCAAS is still used where DIAAS data is missing.

PDCAAS

The PDCAAS was the gold standard method for determining protein quality used by the Food and Agriculture Organization (FAO) of the United Nations (UN) for 20 years between 1993 and 2013[7]. The PDCAAS evaluates a food's protein quality by comparing the amount of essential amino acids that are within a food source to a reference protein (usually eggs). *PDCAAS values are given a score of between 0 and 1.0*. Proteins that score above 1.0 are capped at 1.0. This has always been a major limitation of the PDCAAS and does not give a clear differentiation between protein types of varying quality[8]. For example, the PDCAAS for Whole Milk Protein and Soy Protein are both 1.0, whereas the DIAAS values are equivalent to 1.43 (Excellent) & 0.92 (Good), which better highlights the drastic difference in their quality.

DIAAS

The DIAAS is the most up-to-date method for determining protein quality adopted by the FAO of the UN in 2013.[9] The DIAAS more accurately reflects the true nutritional value and quality of proteins in both isolated and mixed sources. The DIAAS test generates 9 values (compared to the PDCAAS's 1 value) per protein or protein blend and the lowest score is used to reflect the quality of the protein/protein blend. Unlike the PDCAAS the scoring of the DIAAS can exceed 100% as *the 100% value is used as a marker of excellent/ high-quality proteins* and an optimal provider of dietary essential amino acids. *A DIAAS value of between 75% and 99% represents a good quality protein*, but does not provide an optimal supply of essential amino acids. *DIAAS values of <75% are low/suboptimal proteins* and cannot use any claims to its protein quality. Overleaf is a table showing the DIAAS values for some commonly used protein sources and their respective quality.

BIOAVAILABILITY

PROTEIN SOURCE	DIAAS (%)	QUALITY
Whole Milk Powder	143	Excellent / Optimal
Milk Protein Concentrate	118	Excellent / Optimal
Whole Milk	114	Excellent / Optimal
Egg - Hard Boiled	113	Excellent / Optimal
Beef	111	Excellent / Optimal
Whey Protein Isolate	109	Excellent / Optimal
Chicken Breast	108	Excellent / Optimal
Soy Protein Concentrate	98.5	Good
Whey Protein Concentrate	98.3	Good
Pea Protein	91.5	Good
Soy Protein	91.5	Good
Soy Protein Isolate	90	Good
Chickpeas	83	Good
Pea Protein Concentrate	82	Good
Mixed Diet: Wheat, Peas, and Whole Milk Powder	82	Good
Rice (Cooked)	59	Low / Suboptimal
Peas (Cooked)	58	Low / Suboptimal
Rye	47.6	Low / Suboptimal
Wheat	40.2	Low / Suboptimal
Almonds	40	Low / Suboptimal
Rice Protein Concentrate	37	Low / Suboptimal
Corn-Based Cereal	10	Low / Suboptimal

Adapted from MondoScience.com, (2020)[10]

Despite these protein quality assessment methods being an invaluable tool, PDCAAS or DIAAS values are rarely included on food packaging due to the high costs of conducting the tests. A low DIAAS value does not mean you cannot use this as a source of protein, rather it informs you that this source cannot meet your protein needs alone and may need other sources to help meet all your essential amino acids needs.

Practical Applications

How to Improve Micronutrient Absorption

Optimising the bioavailability of your diet starts with how you source, store, and prepare your food. Here are 6 tips on shopping, food prep, and storage that will maximise the nutrients in your food[11]:

1. **Eat Local / Grow Your Own** - Where possible try to eat crops from local farms or even try growing a few items in your garden or planters. By minimising the distance your food has taken you decrease the loss of nutrients that occurs from the time they're picked to when they're on your plate.
2. **Chop, Crush, Blend, and Soak** - Chopping up your fruits and vegetables helps to breakdown the tough plant cell walls making them easier to digest. Crushing items like garlic and onions helps to release alliinase, an enzyme that aids the phytonutrient allicin. Soaking grains and beans reduces phytic acid levels which can block the absorption of iron, calcium, magnesium, and zinc.
3. **Properly Store Your Foods** - Some foods like to be kept cool while others prefer room temperature. All non-root vegetables should be stored in the fridge. All fruits (including avocados and tomatoes) and root vegetables should be kept at room temperature and away from direct light. Storing cut fruit and vegetables with slices of lemon/lime or citrus juice will slow their decay.
4. **Minimise Cooking Heat Sensitive Nutrients** - Water-soluble vitamins (i.e. B Vitamins and Vitamin C), are best absorbed when eaten raw or when prepared through techniques that minimise nutrient loss. For these foods try blanching, steaming, sautéing, roasting, and/or microwaving rather than boiling.
5. **Some Foods Are Better Cooked** - The bioavailability of the phytonutrients lycopene and beta-carotene are greatly increased from cooking. Iron and other minerals also benefit from cooking as it reduces oxalates and other anti-nutrients which inhibit absorption. Protein in eggs and meat also greatly increases bioavailability by denaturing the protein which makes them easier to digest.
6. **Frozen Veggies Are A Good Option** - Many people will avoid frozen foods in favour of fresh. However, most frozen vegetables are frozen shortly after picking and retain much higher levels of essential nutrients when compared to some fresh produce which may have taken weeks to reach your plate.

Not all of the 29 micronutrients suffer from poor bioavailability with some present in good amounts in a diverse and healthy diet alone. However, there are a few that do require a helping hand and a little extra planning. The easiest way to is to combine foods which are rich in bioavailability enhancers and try to avoid combining foods which inhibit bioaviability. This is easier than it sounds and I have detailed some simple ways to achieve this below.

Bioavailability-Enhancing Food Combinations

Fat-Soluble Vitamins (i.e. Vitamin A, D, E, & K) with 3 - 5 g of fat per meal - Because fat-soluble vitamins are stored in fat and travel within your body inside fat molecules, it helps to eat some fat with fat-soluble vitamins to ensure they can be transported effectively[12]. Examples include eating cooked tomatoes with olive oil, pairing guacamole with salsa, or dipping carrots in hummus.

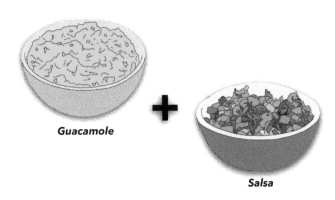

Guacamole

Salsa

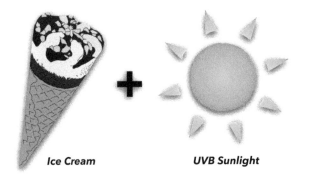

Ice Cream   *UVB Sunlight*

Calcium with Vitamin D - Both of these nutrients aid in the absorption of the other[13] and some dairy products are now fortified with Vitamin D as a result. Good options to try are pairing salmon with spinach, or my personal favourite some tasty ice cream while enjoying the sunshine.

Calcium with Inulin - Covered in detail in the next chapter, inulin is a prebiotic that you feed the good bacteria living in your gut. The healthier and more diverse they are, the better you can absorb valuable nutrients from your diet. Calcium is particularly aided by this effect[14] so try eating spinach or kale with garlic, or milk / yoghurt with bananas.

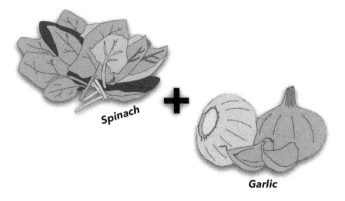

Spinach

Garlic

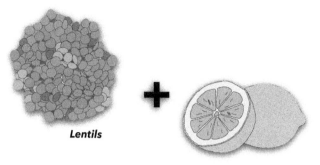

Lentils

Lemon Juice

Non-Haem Iron with Vitamin C - Squeezing some lemon juice over spinach or lentils, adding fruits to your breakfast cereal, or enjoying a glass of fruit juice with an iron-rich meal can all help to increase non-haem iron absorption[15].

Non-Haem Iron with Haem Iron - Haem iron is not only more bioavailable than non-haem iron it aids in the absorption of non-haem iron as well[16]. Therefore, eating your meat or fish with some leafy greens can give you an extra boost in dietary iron.

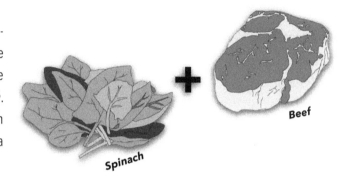

Beef

Spinach

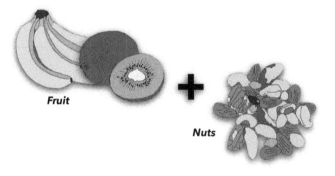

Fruit

Nuts

Vitamin C with Vitamin E - These vitamins both help with the absorption of the other and are easily combined by eating fruits and nuts together[17]. This can be enjoyed on their own as a healthy snack or added to salads as a topping.

Vitamin B12 & Folate (Vitamin B9) - B Vitamins like to work together and aid in the absorption of each other[18]. For meat-eaters, this is easily achieved as most meat sources are rich in B Vitamins. For vegetarians and vegans, however, you are best taking a Vitamin B complex supplement or B12 supplements with fortified cereals and grains.

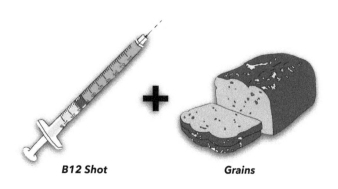

B12 Shot

Grains

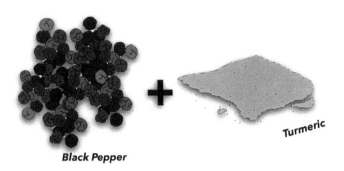

Black Pepper

Turmeric

Turmeric with Black Pepper - Turmeric has been used around the world for centuries and has seen a surge in popularity in recent years due to its anti-inflammatory and anti-oxidant properties. Black pepper makes the curcumin in turmeric more bioavailable[19] and is easily eaten together in curry dishes like Tarka Dal.

Bioavailability-Inhibiting Food Combinations

Inhibiting food combinations may affect your daily requirements of key nutrients. In can be difficult to assess the exact amount inhibiting combinations may limit absorption so it is best practice to try to avoid known combinations that have been shown to have a significant effect on absorption. However, the inhibitory effect of some anti-nutrients can be used to your advantage to limit the amount of harmful compounds you absorb.

Calcium, Iron, and Zinc with Phytic Acid - Phytic acid is abundant in plant foods including wholegrains, cereals, nuts, seeds, and beans. To reduce the phytic acid in these foods try soaking or fermenting them. The effects of phytic acid on inhibiting nutrient absorption are stronger when using supplements[20]. Therefore, if you are taking calcium, iron, and/or zinc supplements try to take them at a separate time to meals high in phytic acid.

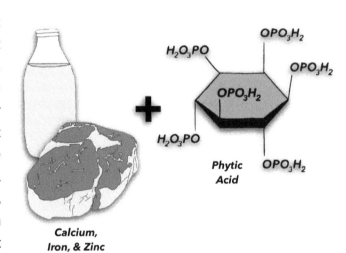

Calcium, Iron, & Zinc

Phytic Acid

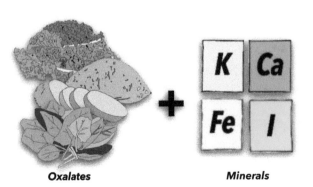

Oxalates

Minerals

Oxalates (a.k.a. Oxalic Acid) with Minerals - Oxalates are in high concentration in rhubarb, spinach, beetroot, kale, peanuts, and sweet potatoes. The oxalates in these healthy foods can be reduced by 30 - 90% through boiling[21] but are a greater concern for those with kidney issues.

Phytosterols with Saturated Fats - Phytosterols are extracted from plant foods and often added to spreads and fermented milk drinks. The phytosterols prevent cholesterol from being absorbed in the gut and can have benefi cial effects in lowering cardiovascular disease risk[22].

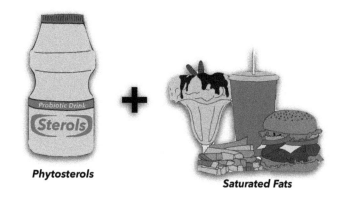

Phytosterols

Saturated Fats

Improving the Bioavailability of Plant-Based Proteins

Animal sources of protein are complete proteins and are extremely bioavailable. However, plant sources of protein are incomplete proteins and have much lower levels of bioavailability when eating from a single source. Therefore, if you are a vegetarian or vegan your sources of high quality protein are much lower and careful diet planning is needed to prevent any potential deficiencies. Below are 5 tips for vegetarians/vegans to help optimise their protein bioavailability[23].

1. **Vary your protein sources over the day** - By eating different sources of proteins within a meal and/or over the course of the day you help increase the bioavailability of your total protein intake and fi ll in any missing gaps in your essential amino acid intake.
2. **Consider increasing your daily protein intake** - Due to the decreased bioavailability of plant proteins you may benefi t from increasing your protein intake to 2.0 - 2.5 g/kg/day. This is more important if your diet has little variety and not following tip number 1.
3. **Eat fibre with your protein** - Fibre is a great source of prebiotics (See Chapter 6) that take care of your gut microbiome. If your gut bacteria are thriving they help you to extract more valuable nutrients from your food, including protein.
4. **Try protein supplements** - Protein supplements may be absorbed more easily than whole foods particularly if they include protein blends. This can be an effective way to meet your daily protein requirements and also increase bioavailability.
5. **(Vegetarians Only) eat eggs and/or dairy twice a day** - As your best source of protein try to have 2 - 3 portions of dairy (e.g. milk, cheese, yoghurt) and/or eggs per day. As a reminder, almond, oat, and soya milks do not contain any dairy.

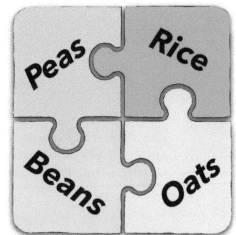

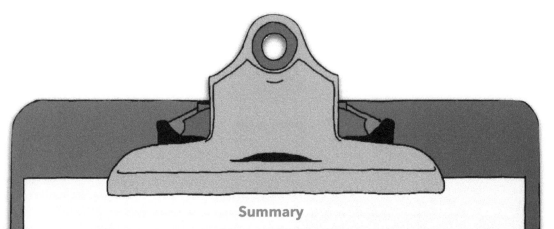

Summary

✓ The food and drink you consume is affected by several factors that determine how much of the nutrients within are absorbed and utilised by your body. This process is known as **bioavailability**.

✓ The nutrients within your food/drink bind together into a chemical structure called a matrix. **Nutrients are released from the matrix and made available for use through chewing and digestive enzymes**.

✓ Some nutrients aid in the absorption of other nutrient and are called **Bio-Enhancers**. Conversely, some nutrients hinder the absorption of other nutrients and these are called **Bio-Inhibitors**.

✓ Bioavailability affects all macro- and micronutrients but has a much greater effect on micronutrients.

✓ The bioavailability of protein is assessed using 2 main digestibility tests, called the **Protein Digestibility Corrected Amino Acid Score (PDCAAS)** and the gold standard test the **Digestibility Indispensable Amino Acid Score (DIAAS)**.

✓ How you purchase, store, and prepare your foods can affect how many nutrients remain in your food before you come to eat them.

✓ **Fat-soluble vitamins are more easily absorbed when eaten with fat**.

✓ **Calcium absorption can be helped by Vitamin D and Inulin**. Calcium returns the favour by helping more Vitamin D to be absorbed.

✓ **Non-Haem Iron absorption is added by Vitamin C and Haem Iron**.

✓ **B Vitamins like to work together and aid each other to be absorbed**. A key combination is B12 with Folate (Vitamin B9).

✓ **Turmeric with Black Pepper is a helpful combination that aids with inflammation and reducing free radical activity**.

✓ **Phytic Acid in grains, beans, seeds, nuts, and cereals can inhibit the absorption of Calcium, Iron, and Zinc**. Soaking or fermenting phytic acid rich foods can help reduce its effects on nutrient absorption.

✓ **Oxalates found in rhubarb, spinach, sweet potato, kale, and peanuts may inhibit the absorption of minerals**. Boiling these foods can reduce oxalates by 30 - 90%.

✓ **Phytosterols found in certain spreads and fermented milk drinks can help reduce the absorption of dietary cholesterol** and reduce your risk of cardiovascular disease.

✓ Plant-based proteins are poorly absorbed on their own and **varying your plant proteins, eating more fibre, and using supplements can all help to increase protein bioavailability**.

REFERENCES

[1] Heaney RP (2001). *Factors influencing the measurement of bioavailability, taking calcium as a model*. Journal of Nutrition 131(suppl):1344S-1348S.

[2] The European Food International Council, (2010), *Nutrient bioavailability: Getting the most out of food*, Retrieved from https://www.eufic.org/en/food-today/article/nutrient-bioavailability-getting-the-most-out-of-food

[3] Precision Nutrition, (2020), *10 ways to get the most nutrients from your food*, Retrieved from https://www.precisionnutrition.com/10-ways-to-get-the-most-nutrients

[4] Grand, R. J., Watkins, J. B., and Torti, F. M., (1976), *Development of the Human Gastrointestinal Tract: A Review*, Gastroenterology, 70, 790-810

[5] Rein, M. J., Renouf, M., Cruz-Hernandez, C., Actis-Goretta, L., Thakkar, S. K., and da Silva Pinto, M., (2013), *Bioavailability of bioactive food compounds: a challenging journey of bioefficacy*, British Journal of Clinical Pharmacology, 75(3), 588-602, https://dx.doi.org/10.1111%2Fj.1365-2125.2012.04425.x

[6] UK Statutory Instruments, *The Bread and Flour Regulations 1998*, Retrieved from http://www.legislation.gov.uk/uksi/1998/141/contents/made

[7] Boutrif, E., (1991), Food Quality and Consumer Protection Group, Food Policy and Nutrition Division, FAO, Rome: "*Recent Developments in Protein Quality Evaluation*" Food, Nutrition and Agriculture, Issue 2/3, http://www.fao.org/docrep/U5900t/u5900t07.htm

[8] Schaafsma, G., (2012), *Advantages and limitations of the protein digestibility-corrected amino acid score (PDCAAS) as a method for evaluating protein quality in human diets*, British Journal of Nutrition, 108, Supplement 2, S333-336, https://doi.org/10.1017/S0007114512002541

[9] Food and Agriculture Organization of the United Nations, (2011), *Dietary protein quality evaluation in human nutrition*, Rterieved from http://www.fao.org/ag/humannutrition/35978-02317b979a686a57aa4593304ffc17f06.pdf

[10] MondoScience, (2020), *100% Amino Acid Score*, Retrieved from https://www.mondoscience.com/blog/2017/10/25/100-amino-acid-score

[11] Precision Nutrition, (2020), *10 ways to get the most nutrients from your food*, Retrieved from https://www.precisionnutrition.com/10-ways-to-get-the-most-nutrients

[12] Albahrani, A. A., and Greaves, R. F., (2016), *Fat-Soluble Vitamins: Clinical Indications and Current Challenges for Chromatographic Measurement*, The Clinical Biochemist - Reviews, 37(1), 27-47,

[13] Christakos, S., Dhawan, P., Porta, A., Mady, L. J., and Seth, T., (2011), *Vitamin D and Intestinal Calcium Absorption*, Molecular and Cellular Endocrinology, 347(1-2), 25-29, https://doi.org/10.1016/j.mce.2011.05.038

[14] Shah, M., Chandalia, M., Adams-Huet, B., Brinkley, L. J., Sakhaee, K., Grundy, S. M., and Garg, A., (2009), *Effect of a Hugh-Fiber Diet Compared With a Moderate-Fiber Diet on Calcium and Other Mineral Balances in Subjects With Type 2 Diabetes*, Diabetes Care, 32(6), 990-995, https://dol.org/10.2337/dc09-0126

[15] Cook, J., D., and Reddy, M. B., (2001), *Effect of ascorbic acid intake on non heme-iron absorption from a complete diet,* American Journal of Clinical Nutrition, 73(1), 93-98, https://doi.org/10.1093/ajcn/73.1.93

[16] Hurrell R & Egli I (2010). *Iron bioavailability and dietary reference values*. American Journal of Clinical Nutrition. https://doi.org/10.3945/ajcn.2010.28674F

[17] Reboul E. (2017). *Vitamin E Bioavailability: Mechanisms of Intestinal Absorption in the Spotlight*. Antioxidants (Basel, Switzerland), 6(4), 95. https://doi.org/10.3390/antiox6040095

[18] O'Leary, F., and Samman, S., (2010), *Vitamin B12 in Health and Disease*, Nutrients, 2(3), 299-316, https://doi.org/10.3390/nu2030299

[19] Trujillo, J., Chirino, Y. I., Molina-Jijón, E., Andérica-Romero, A. C., Tapia, E., and Pedraza-Chaverrí, J., (2013), *Renoprotective effect of the antioxidant curcumin: Recent findings*, Redox Biology, 1(1), 448-456, https://doi.org/10.1016/j.redox.2013.09.003

[20] Zhou, J. R., and Erdman Jr., J. W., (1995). *Phytic acid in health and disease*. Critical Reviews in Food Science and Nutrition 35(6):495-508.

[21] Heaney, R. P., & Weaver, C. M. (1989). *Oxalate: effect on calcium absorbability*. The American journal of clinical nutrition, 50(4), 830–832. https://doi.org/10.1093/ajcn/50.4.830

[22] Demonty I, et al. (2009). *Continuous dose-response relationship of the LDL-cholesterol-lowering effect of phytosterol intake*. Journal of Nutrition 139(2):271-284.

[23] Third Wave Nutrition, (2020), *A Guide to Vegan Protein*, Retrieved from https://thirdwavenutrition.com/blogs/news/a-guide-to-vegan-protein

6

THE GUT MICROBIOME

What is the gut microbiome, what does it do and why should you care about it?

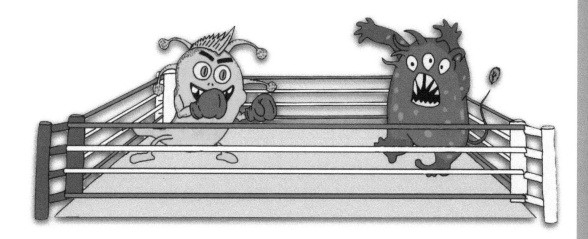

Your ability to digest and utilise key nutrients, maintain a healthy weight, reduce your risk of disease and more, is significantly affected by the trillions of bacteria that live within your digestive tract[1]. The environment these trillions of helpful bacteria create within your digestive tract is called your *Gut Microbiome*. It is worth mentioning early on that your gut microbiome is not all bacteria as it also contains many yeasts, parasites, protozoa, viruses, and archaea. However, to date, the majority of the research conducted has been done on gut bacteria and therefore the potential effects these other organisms play on your health may currently be underestimated[2].

What Is The Gut Microbiome?

Your gut microbiome (***biome*** = a large community of living organisms) acts like a "virtual organ" that lives mostly in your large intestine and with similar amounts of metabolic activity as your liver or kidneys[3]. This virtual organ is essential in the development of your immune system, central nervous system, gastrointestinal system (***gastro*** = belly), and plays a role in your metabolism, particularly in glucose and weight management (although this is not yet fully understood)[4]. Your gut microbiome is a colony of 100 trillion microorganisms weighing roughly 1.5 kg and contains more than 150 times the number of genes than human genes in your body[5]. There are over 500 different species of gut microbiota and they have an enormous effect on your overall health and performance. Each human being has around 150 species of gut bacteria, with a unique diversity of microorganisms and varying different amounts of both "good" and "bad" bacteria. Just like fingerprints, even identical twins have different gut microbiomes despite being genetically identical due to the individual way each person interacts with the world around them[6].

Your gut microbiome is how you interact with the outside world and starts with microbial exposure from drinking the amniotic fluid (i.e. the "water" you live in while in the womb), and from transfers from your mother's microbiome via the placenta[7,8]. This transfer of microbiota continues when you are born and you are exposed to numerous types of microorganisms from your mother's cervix, vagina, and perineum[9]. This transfer continues further with breastfeeding and forms the initial basis of your unique gut microbiome. While this may sound a little gross to some, baby's need to be exposed to and live in symbiosis with these microorganisms. Children who are born via caesarean-section, spend large amounts of time in hospital after birth; receive large amounts of antibiotics, or are bottle-fed, may miss out on these natural experiences and often have more health issues due to not developing a bifidobacterium dominant gut microbiome[10].

99% of your gut bacteria are anaerobic organisms (**anaerobic** = work without oxygen) and are dominated by 2 divisions: *Firmicutes* (firmis = strong, cutis = skin, referring to their thick cell membranes) and *Bacteroidetes* (bacterie = small staff, dete = fingers, referring to their rod-like appearance). Firmicutes comprise around 64% of your gut microbiome and bacteroidetes around 23%. The remaining gut microbiota is comprised of Actinobacteria, Proteobacteria, Fusobacteria, and Verrucomicrobia. Your gut microbiome and mitochondria (your body's energy cells) communicate with each other via cell signalling. This inter-cell communication allows the bacteria, fungi, yeasts, and other cells to effectively communicate with each other to positively impact your health by influencing energy production, reducing inflammation, and improving your gut barrier[11]. Each individual will have a different gut microbiome unique to them, however, people can potentially be separated into different groups based upon the clusters of bacteria that form their microbiome. These clusters are called **Enterotypes** and include *Prevotella*, *Bacteroides*, and *Ruminococcus*. These clustered groupings of gut microbiota are used to study the gut microbiome and determine possible links between certain clusters and disease. Low levels of bacterial diversity of the gut microbiota has been noted in a wide variety of diseases. The more diverse the gut microbiota, the more robust the gut microbiome is against disease and the greater the ability to compensate for any missing species needed to keep the host healthy. Many companies offer enterotype testing, however, before you can properly understand what these tests can tell you, you need to understand a little about the bacteria themselves and what they do in your body.

Good Bacteria

A healthy gut microbiome is a balanced ecosystem which helps to prevent potentially harmful bacteria like Pseudomonas, Proteus, Staphylococci, and Clostridia that can cause pain, infections, diarrhoea/constipation, toxin production, inflammation, and chronic disease[12]. A balanced gut microbiome has potentially helpful bacteria such as *Lactobacilli*, *Eubacteria*, and *Bifidobacteria* that inhibit harmful bacteria, modulate immune functions, aid in digestion/nutrient absorption, stimulate motility, and are involved in synthesising some vitamins[13]. Good bacteria can be divided into lactic acid producing bacteria, non-lactic acid producing bacteria, and non-pathogenic yeasts. The roles of some specific key species are detailed below:

Lactic Acid Bacteria	Non-Lactic Acid Bacteria	Non-Pathogenic Yeasts
Lactobacillus species	Bacillus species	Saccharomyces boulardii
Bifidobacterium species	Proprionibacterium species	
Streptococcus thermophilus	E. Coli Nissle 1917	
Enterococcus faecium		
Lactococcus species		
Leuconostoc species		
Pediococcus species		

Lactobacillus

The lactobacillus family of bacteria provide several general benefits to human health by:

- Producing lactic acid, carbon dioxide, ethanol, and acetic acid.
- Aid in digesting and metabolising proteins and carbohydrates.
- Synthesise some B Vitamins and Vitamin K.
- Catabolise bile salts.
- Enhance innate and acquired immunity.
- Inhibit pro-inflammatory mediators.
- Provide antimicrobial activities against a wide variety of pathogens including E. coli, Staphylococcus, Pseudomonas etc.[14]

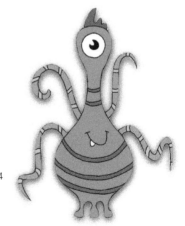

Common Species of Lactobacillus Bacteria		
L. acidophilus	L. fermentum	L. paracasei
L. brevis	L. gasseri	L. plantarum
L. bulgaricus	L. helveticus	L. reuteri
L. casei	L. jensenii	L. rhamnosus
L. crispatus	L. johnsonii	L. salivarius

L. = Lactobacillus

Lactobacillus acidophilus is possibly the most well-known probiotic found in kefir and sauerkraut and sometimes miso, yoghurts, and tempeh. L. acidophilus is only present in the gut microbiome when actively ingested in the diet (a.k.a. **transient bacteria**) and helps to breakdown casein and gluten; ferments lactose; some simple sugars and polysaccharides, and reduces the concentration of carcinogenic enzymes within the gut microbiome[15].

Lactobacillus rhamnosus is one of the most well-studied probiotics and is often found in a variety of foods, such as dairy products. L. rhamnosus is a fragile and transient species that enhances innate and acquired immunity, inhibits pro-inflammatory cytokines, and aids in the digestion of dairy products through the production of the enzyme lactase. L. rhamnosus is often added to milks, cheeses, yoghurts, and other dairy products to enhance their probiotic content or to aid in cheese ripening to enhance its flavour[16]. Despite L. rhamnosus being commonplace in some foods, it is often not listed in the ingredients list.

Lactobacillus casei is a hardy and adaptive species often used for the treatment of several diseases including Crohn's disease, Irritable Bowel Syndrome (IBS), Inflammatory Bowel Disease (IBD), and lactose intolerance. L. Casei is another transient species that aid human health by decreasing pro-inflammatory cytokines and is needed for dendritic cell differentiation[17]. L. casei is found naturally in yoghurts, yoghurt-like fermented milks, and certain cheeses.

Lactobacillus plantarum is ubiquitous in plants and lacking in most modern diets. L. plantarum is another transient bacteria found in fermented foods like sauerkraut and kimchi. L. plantarum has a high resistance to bile and acid, decreases pro-inflammatory cytokines, facilitates IL-10 and central regularity cytokines, supports intestinal barrier function, and reduces translocation of gut flora[18].

Bifidobacterium

The bifidobacterium family of bacteria are a fastidious, Y-shaped species that works strictly anaerobically. Reduced populations of bifidobacterium is associated with increased disease prevalence/poor health and robust populations are associated with better gut and immune health by:

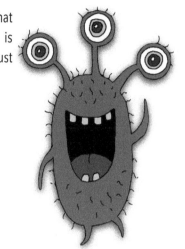

- Metabolising lactose.
- Fermenting non-digestible oligosaccharides.
- Synthesising B vitamins and vitamin K.
- Enhance innate and acquired immunity.
- Inhibit pro-inflammatory mediators.
- Inhibit pathogens via organic acids and hydrogen peroxide[19].

Common Species of Bifidobacterium		
B. adolescents	B. breve	B. longum
B. animalis	B. infantis	B. thermophilum
B. bifidum	B. lactis	

B. = Bifidobacterium

Bifidobacterium longum often the dominant form of gut bifidobacterium, B. longum ferments an array of oligosaccharides, is resistant to bile salts, inhibits enterotoxigenic E. Coli receptor binding and translocation, inhibits clostridium proliferation, aids in reducing dietary allergies, and modulates cytokine response to respiratory antigens. Almost double the amount of B. longum is found in the guts of elite athletes compared to recreational athletes/healthy individuals suggesting a positive relationship between increased physical activity and a healthy gut microbiome[20]. B. longum is found in several food sources including kefir, yoghurt, goats cheese, seaweed (kelp), and miso.

Bifidobacterium bifidum is often reduced in infants who suffer from more allergic reactions and B. bifidum populations naturally decline with age. B. bifidum protects against allergies and enhances immunity. B. bifidum is used in the treatment of several diseases including IBS and restoring the intestinal barrier following chemotherapy, lung infections, diarrhoea and more[21]. B. bifidum is found in cultured yoghurts, cured meats, sauerkraut, sourdough bread, kimchi, tempeh, miso, kefir, and buttermilk.

Bifidobacterium infantis is a common type of gut bacteria in infants but rarely frequent in adults. B. infantis suppresses bacteroides vulgatus, improves cytokines ratios in IBS sufferers, promotes normal microbiota in children with diarrhoea, and along with L. Acidophilus reduces risk of necrotising enterocolitis in very low birth weight infants[22].

Bifidobacterium breve reduces bacteroides fragilis and C. perfringens populations; improves weight gain in low birth weight infants; is resistant to bile acid, pepsin, and pancreatin; enhances B cell antibody production, and eliminates campylobacter jejuni (a common cause of bacterial infection)[23]. B. breve can be found in kombucha, sauerkraut, and kefir.

Bifidobacterium animalis like B. longum, B. animalis is present in much higher levels in the gut of elite athletes[24]. Found in fermented milk, yoghurt, and soy products, B. animalis is used to treat IBS, diarrhoea, yeast infections, lactose intolerance, urinary tract infections, and eczema[25].

Bacillus

Bacillus are fermentation end products that include lactate, acetate, ethanol, acetoin, and 2,3-butanediol. Used in traditional fermented fish, manioc, and soy foods these transient commensals aid in human health by:

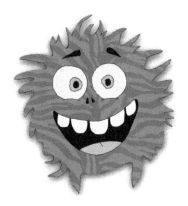

- Enhancing innate and acquired immunity.
- Inhibit pathogens via bacteriocins and lipopeptides.
- Promote colonocyte health via heat shock proteins.
- Aid in the treatment of IBS and antibiotic-associated diarrhoea.[26]

Common Species of Bacillus Bacteria		
B. cereus	B. laterosporus	B. subtilis
B. clausii	B. licheniformis	
B. coagulans	B. pumilus	

B. = Bacillus

Streptococcus Thermophilus

S. thermophilus is a transient species that is used in food production as a yoghurt and cheese starter[27]. S. thermophilus is well adapted to lactose and produces antibiotic like chemicals that help prevent infection from clostridium difficile and pneumonia by preventing pathogen proliferation. S. thermophilus also reduces DNA damage to premalignant legions, protects against pathogenic streptococcus, and is used in the treatment of ulcerative colitis and rotavirus[28].

Saccharomyces Boulardii

S. boulardii is a transient, non-pathogenic yeast that is most commonly used for treating diarrhoea caused by gastrointestinal overgrowth by bad bacteria or caused by antibiotics[29]. S. boulardii is the active ingredient in Asian medicinal teas and is both heat and pH resistant. S. boulardii increases the gut production of short-chain fatty acids, protects against protein-based dietary allergies, and inhibits certain toxins[30].

Probiotics & Prebiotics

Probiotics

Probiotics have been a part of human nutrition for thousands of years as they are found naturally in fruits and vegetables. The concentration of probiotics within the human diet increased significantly from circa 10,000 BCE with the introduction of fermented food and drinks. Fermentation is a traditional way to increase the 'shelf-life' of stored foods to prevent them from spoiling. In the modern world, fermented foods have seen a drastic decline since the invention of refrigerators. Dairy products, most notably yoghurt are another great source of probiotics and have formed part of the human diet since circa 3,000 BCE. Yoghurt is a good source of probiotics to those with lactose intolerance as yoghurt is naturally low in lactose and aids in the digestion of lactose-containing dairy foods such as milk and cheese[31]. Examples of traditional high probiotics yoghurts include Skyr from Iceland and Kefir from Eastern Europe. Unfortunately, probiotics are rarely listed on ingredients lists but are a crucial part in the production of many cheeses, yoghurts, and fermented foods. Despite claims made by questionable Netflix 'documentaries' dairy consumption is extremely beneficial to human health with links to reducing type 2 diabetes risk, cardiovascular disease risk, hypertension, and inflammation as well as improving the gut barrier and potentially aiding in weight maintenance.

The term probiotics was first defined in 1965 as *"growth-promoting factors produced by microbes that promote the flourishing of good microbes that live in symbiosis with their host and provides benefits to human health"*.[32] However, the so-called godfather of probiotics wrote about the gut microbiome long before this in his 1907 book "The Prolongation of Life" where he stated that *"the dependence of the intestinal microbes on the food [we eat] makes it possible to adopt measures to modify the flora in our bodies and replace the harmful microbes with useful microbes"*.[33] The benefits of certain food sources on health has been documented as far back as the Ancient Greek philosopher Hippocrates (*circa 460 - 370 BC*), who famously said *"all disease begins in the gut"* and recommended the consumption of sour milk to improve longevity. In the modern world, probiotics can be used in the treatment of diarrhoea, inflammatory bowel disease (including ulcerative. colitis, Crohn's disease, and pouchitis), IBS, vaginal dysbiosis (including bacterial vaginosis and urinary tract infections), allergies, eczema, dermatitis, lactose intolerance, hyperlipidaemia, and more.

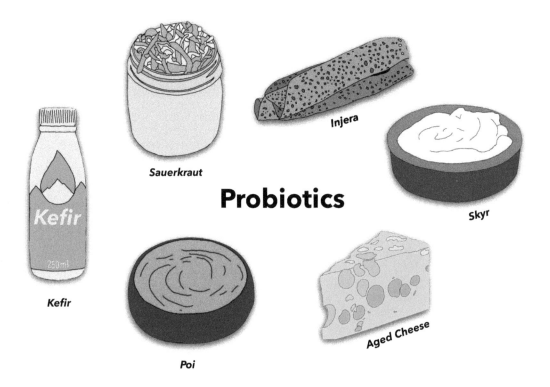

Injera

Sauerkraut

Probiotics

Skyr

Kefir

Aged Cheese

Poi

The potential benefits of probiotics in your diet are astonishing with research showing that probiotics may help IBS symptoms by modulating pain receptors, specifically the opioid and cannabinoid receptors with similar performance to taking morphine[34]. Human trials looking at the effects of probiotics on the gut-brain axis have shown that probiotics may also improve autism symptoms and Alzheimer's. Communication between your brain and gut works both ways with stress causing a breakdown of the bacteria-containing mucus layer in the gut and breaks the gut barrier layer. This helps to explain why IBS/IBD sufferers may often have flare-ups in symptoms during periods of heightened stress and may find traditional diet only approaches to managing these conditionings (i.e. low-FODMAP diets) ineffective. Probiotics also 'harvest' around 10-15% of the calories in the fibre your eat, however, excess calorie extraction from dietary fibre may increase obesity risk if certain negative forms of gut bacteria are present in higher amounts. An imbalance in your gut microbiome is called Dysbiosis and has been linked to several health conditions including multiple sclerosis and rheumatoid arthritis.

Prebiotics

Prebiotics are defined as *"non-digestible substances that stimulate the growth and/or metabolic activity of select gut microbes leading to human health benefits"*.[35] The main source of prebiotics is dietary fibre that are found naturally in fruit, vegetables, pulses, legumes, and grains. However, not all fibre is prebiotic as some are digested more by your probiotics than others. This does not mean the other types of fibre serve no purpose as they also help with creating bulk to your stools which aids in nutrients passing through your digestive tract at the correct speed and making your bowel movement healthier. It is possible to take supplements of prebiotics as well as probiotic supplements, however, as always, you should always follow a food first approach and focus first on increasing your whole food sources of prebiotics before you consider possible supplementation. Examples of whole foods which are naturally high in prebiotics are asparagus, garlic, chicory root, Jerusalem artichokes, wheat, honey, barley, bananas, tomatoes, rye, cow's milk, peas, beans, and seaweed. The easiest way to think about probiotics are prebiotics is that probiotics are helpful bacteria you need to regularly eat to keep you in good health. You then need to eat plenty of prebiotics to feed your probiotics so then can reproduce and flourish within your gut.

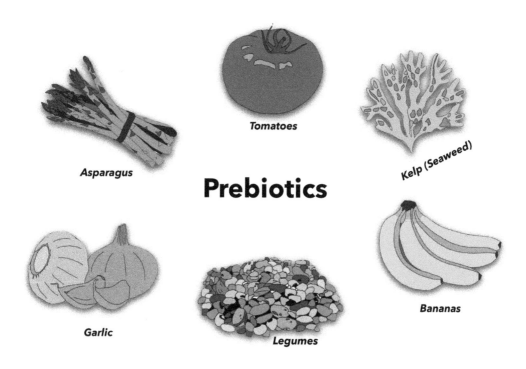

Tomatoes

Kelp (Seaweed)

Asparagus

Prebiotics

Garlic

Legumes

Bananas

A less frequently used term is **synbiotics**, which are foods or supplements that contain both pre- and probiotic properties (e.g. kimchi or yoghurt with whole fruits).

Practical Applications

Optimising Your Gut Microbiome

The more diverse the community of bacteria in your gut, the healthier you are and the more resilient you are to chronic disease. While experts agree that your diet is the largest influencer on your gut microbiome, your food environment still plays a significant role. It has been suggested that your gut microbiome has become less diverse due to the lack of exposure to soil and dirt (both from our food and exposure to nature); a lack of fermented foods (due to more advanced refrigeration techniques), the increase in dietary sugar and processed food consumption, and the overuse of antibiotics in medicine and livestock feed. To improve your gut microbiome, several techniques can be employed collectively known as modulation. You can modulate your gut microbiome in both positive and negative ways through your diet, supplementation, antibiotics, and faecal transplants. Increasing the diversity of your diet and supplementation are both ways of trying to modulate your gut microbiome through the use of Probiotics and Prebiotics. As always, the best approach to improving your health and performance should be a food first mindset and it is recommended to follow these 8 tips to improve your gut microbiome:

1. **Consume 30 different types of plants per week** - This includes fruit, vegetables, grains, beans, pulses, legumes, nuts, and seeds. Aim to eat a wide variety of options including lots of different colours. This will increase your fibre intake and sources of prebiotics as well as your vitamin and mineral intake.

2. **Increase your intake of fermented foods** - Fermented foods are found in traditional cuisine from all around the world and include Poi (Hawaii), Pozol (Mexico), Guarapo (Columbia), Champus (Peru), Kimchi (Korea), Natto (Japan), Jun (Tibet), Lassi (India), Injera (Ethiopia), Ayib (Ethiopia), Incwancwa (South Africa), Iru (Nigeria), Sauerkraut (Germany), Smetana (Eastern Europe), Skyr (Iceland), and Kefir (Central Europe).

3. **Reduce your intake of processed and convenience foods** - As a good rule the fewer ingredients listed on the back of the packaging the better. Alternatively, when in a supermarket, primarily select foods from the edges of the store and not the centre. Most supermarkets are laid out with the snacks and junk foods in the aisles near the centre and the fresh produce around the outside.

4. **Stay well hydrated** - Good hydration along with fibre is essential to healthy digestion and to ensure your stools move through your bowels at the appropriate speed. Without this, you do not have enough time for your gut microbiota to absorb valuable nutrients to keep them and you in good health.

5. **Practice good sleep hygiene** - Your gut bacteria need sleep just like you do. Maintaining a healthy circadian rhythm will help maintain the health of your gut microbiome. There are 3 main areas of focus for sleep health: quantity, quality, and consistency. Therefore, try to sleep 7 - 9 hours/night, reduce factors that reduce sleep quality (i.e. smoking, alcohol, caffeine use, etc.), and have a set bedtime and wake time every day of the week.

6. **Stay physically active** - In addition to all the more well-known physical, mental and emotional benefits of exercise, exercise also stimulates a health gut microbiome balance so try to maintain a minimum of 150 minutes of moderate (or harder) exercise per week.

7. **Do not overuse antibiotics** - Antibiotics are a lifesaving invention that are essential for the treatment of bacterial infections. However, antibiotics cannot help with viral infections like the common cold, influenza, and coronavirus so taking them in this situation is pointless. Antibiotics also damage your gut microbiome and decrease short-chain fatty acid production. Therefore, prolonged or unnecessary antibiotics use may impede your resistance to disease and your ability to recover from illness.

8. **Manage your stress levels** - The connection between your gut and your brain (a.k.a the gut-brain axis) is a 2-way street. Periods of increased stress can increase the incidence of digestive discomfort and a poor diet may increase your likelihood of poor mental/emotional wellbeing. Stress is unavoidable but it can manageable. Try to practice mindfulness meditation, keep a journal, employ cognitive behaviour therapy (CBT) techniques, try a relaxing hobby, read, listen to music, or talk with your friends and colleagues. The important thing is to find your way of "switching off" from your daily stressors and better manage your stress levels.

Gut Testing

Do-It-Yourself kits for assessing the health of your gut microbiome are now available from several companies including Atlas Biomed, Chuckling Goat, and Viome. These home testing options involve registering for a kit online, providing a stool sample, then returning the kit via post. The sample you provide is then analysed and the results provided to you via an online portal within a few weeks. These easy-to-use kits can help you to understand your gut microbiome and show which species of bacteria are dominant known as your enterotype. The level of detail provided within these results are quite good but are not as detailed as those provided by more professional services used by nutritionists/dieticians. From your results, these services will often give recommendations on what you can do to modulate your gut microbiome much like the guidance I have provided above. If you are having some digestive issues or find you have a history of potential intolerances to certain foods then a detailed gut microbiome test completed by a registered nutritionist/dietician would be a good idea. However, if you have a more passing interest or are just looking to optimise your health as much as possible then these home testing kit options may be a better choice or save your money just follow the advice above instead. A final word of caution is to remain sceptical about the level of claims some of these services may make from their results. While there is a lot of promising data relating your gut microbiome to health and disease, this is far from conclusive and maybe only a small part of the overall picture.

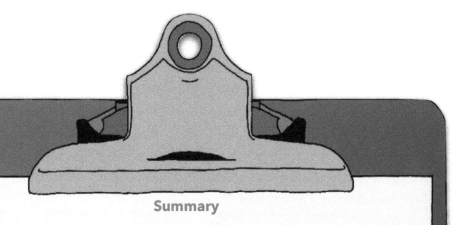

Summary

✓   Your gut microbiome is a type of '**virtual organ**' that is essential in the development of a healthy immune system, central nervous system, gastrointestinal system, and metabolism.

✓   Bacteria, yeasts, parasites, protozoa, viruses, and archaea all work together to make up your unique gut microbiome.

✓   **Your gut microbiome is how you interact with the outside world** and starts when in the womb and accelerated when you are born and exposed to lots of new types of bacteria.

✓   The majority (99%) of your gut bacteria are anaerobic organisms and dominated by 2 divisions: Firmicutes and Bacteroidetes.

✓   Inter-cell communication between your gut microbiome and your body's energy cells (mitochondria) impacts your health in both positive and negative ways.

✓   There are a number of 'good bacteria' including **Lactobacilli**, **Eubacteria**, and **Bifidobacteria** that inhibit the effects of harmful bacteria like E. Coli, Pseudomonas, Staphylococci and more.

✓   **Probiotics are growth-promoting factors produced by microbes that promote the flourishing of your gut bacteria and provide you with several health benefits**.

✓   **Prebiotics are types of fibre which you feed you gut microbiota to help them to grow and keep you healthy**.

✓   You can optimise your gut microbiome through changes to your diet, food environment, and faecal transplants.

✓   Your lifestyle behaviours can have a significant impact on your gut microbiome including good quality sleep, staying hydrated, staying physically active, managing your stress levels, and antibiotic use.

✓   Several companies that offer gut testing however, caution should be taken with any recommendations made from these results alone.

REFERENCES

[1] Qin, J., Li, R., Raes, J. *et al.,* (2010), *A human gut microbial gene catalogue established by metagenomic sequencing*. Nature 464, 59–6. https://doi.org/10.1038/nature08821

[2] Sekirov, I., Russell, S. L., Antunes, L. C., & Finlay, B. B. (2010). *Gut microbiota in health and disease.* Physiological reviews, 90(3), 859–904. https://doi.org/10.1152/physrev.00045.2009

[3] Evans, J. M., Morris, L. S., & Marchesi, J. R. (2013). *The gut microbiome: the role of a virtual organ in the endocrinology of the host.* The Journal of endocrinology, 218(3), R37–R47. https://doi.org/10.1530/JOE-13-0131

[4] Davis C. D. (2016). *The Gut Microbiome and Its Role in Obesity.* Nutrition today, 51(4), 167–174. https://doi.org/10.1097/NT.0000000000000167

[5] Qin, J., Li, R., Raes, J. *et al.,* (2010), *A human gut microbial gene catalogue established by metagenomic sequencing.* Nature 464, 59–6. https://doi.org/10.1038/nature08821

[6] Goodrich, J. K., Davenport, E. R., Beaumont, M., Jackson, M. A., Knight, R., Ober, C., Spector, T. D., Bell, J. T., Clark, A. G., & Ley, R. E. (2016). *Genetic Determinants of the Gut Microbiome in UK Twins.* Cell host & microbe, 19(5), 731–743. https://doi.org/10.1016/j.chom.2016.04.017

[7] Rescigno, M., Urbano, M., Valzasina, B. *et al.* (2001), *Dendritic cells express tight junction proteins and penetrate gut epithelial monolayers to sample bacteria.* Nature Immunology, 2, 361–367. https://doi.org/10.1038/86373

[8] Jiménez, E., Marín, M. L., Martín, R., Odriozola, J. M., Olivares, M., Xaus, J., Fernández, L., & Rodríguez, J. M. (2008). *Is meconium from healthy newborns actually sterile?.* Research in microbiology, 159(3), 187–193. https://doi.org/10.1016/j.resmic.2007.12.007

[9] Arboleya, S., Watkins, C., Stanton, C., & Ross, R. P. (2016). *Gut Bifidobacteria Populations in Human Health and Aging.* Frontiers in microbiology, 7, 1204. https://doi.org/10.3389/fmicb.2016.01204

[10] Valdes, A. M., Walter, J., Segal, E., & Spector, T. D., (2018), *Role of Gut Microbiota in Nutrition and Health*, British Medical Journal, 361, https://doi.org/10.1136/bmj.k2179

[11] Kriss, M., Hazleton, K. Z., Nusbacher, N. M., Martin, C. G., & Lozupone, C. A. (2018). *Low diversity gut microbiota dysbiosis: drivers, functional implications and recovery.* Current opinion in microbiology, 44, 34–40. https://doi.org/10.1016/j.mib.2018.07.003

[12] Rowland, I., Gibson, G., Heinken, A., Scott, K., Swann, J., Thiele, I., & Tuohy, K. (2018). *Gut microbiota functions: metabolism of nutrients and other food components.* European journal of nutrition, 57(1), 1–24. https://doi.org/10.1007/s00394-017-1445-8

[13] Nemska, V., Logar, P., Rasheva, T., Sholeva, Z., Georgieva, N., & Danova, S. (2019). *Functional characteristics of lactobacilli from traditional Bulgarian fermented milk products.* Turkish journal of biology = Turk biyoloji dergisi, 43, 148–153. https://doi.org/10.3906/biy-1808-34

[14] Healthline, (2020), *9 Ways Lactobacillus Acidophilus Can Benefit Your Health*, Retrieved from https://www.healthline.com/nutrition/lactobacillus-acidophilus#section2

[15] Healthline, (2020), *Lactobacillus rhamnosus: A Probiotic With Powerful Benefits*, Retrieved from https://www.healthline.com/nutrition/lactobacillus-rhamnosus

[16] Healthline, (2020), *Why You Should Use the Probiotic Lactobacillus Casei*, Retrieved from https://www.healthline.com/health/digestive-health/lactobacillus-casei

[17] Behera, S. S., Ray, R. C., & Zdolec, N. (2018). Lactobacillus plantarum with Functional Properties: An Approach to Increase Safety and Shelf-Life of Fermented Foods. BioMed research international, 2018, 9361614. https://doi.org/10.1155/2018/9361614

[18] O'Callaghan, A., & van Sinderen, D. (2016). *Bifidobacteria and Their Role as Members of the Human Gut Microbiota.* Frontiers in microbiology, 7, 925. https://doi.org/10.3389/fmicb.2016.00925

[19] Wong, C. B., Odamaki, T., and Xiao, J-Z., (2019), *Beneficial effects of Bifidobacterium longum subsp. longum BB536 on human health: Modulation of gut microbiome as the principal action*, Journal of Functional Foods,54, 506-519, https://doi.org/10.1016/j.jff.2019.02.002

[20] Healthline, (2020), *Bifidobacterium Bifidum: Benefits, Side Effects, and More*, Retrieved from https://www.healthline.com/health/bifidobacterium-bifidum

[21] Healthline, (2020), *How to Use the Probiotic Bifidobacterium Infantis*, Retrieved from https://www.healthline.com/health/bifidobacterium-infantis

[22] Bozzi Cionci, N., Baffoni, L., Gaggìa, F., & Di Gioia, D. (2018). *Therapeutic Microbiology: The Role of Bifidobacterium breve as Food Supplement for the Prevention/Treatment of Paediatric Diseases.* Nutrients, 10(11), 1723. https://doi.org/10.3390/nu10111723

[23] O'Donovan, C. M., Madigan, S. M., Garcia-Perez, I., Rankin, A., O'Sullivan, O., and Cotter, P. D., (2020), *Distinct microbiome composition and metabolome exists across subgroups of elite Irish athletes*, Journal of Science and Medicine in Sport, 23(1), 63-68, https://doi.org/10.1016/j.jsams.2019.08.290

[24] WebMD, (2020), *Bifidobacterium Animalis Capsule*, Retrieved from https://www.webmd.com/drugs/2/drug-167122/bifidobacterium-animalis-oral/details

[25] Elshaghabee, F. M. F., Rokana, N., Gulhane, R. D., Sharma, C., and Panwar, H., (2017), *Bacillus As Potential Probiotics: Status, Concerns, and Future Perspectives*, Frontiers in Microbiology, 8, 1490, https://doi.org/10.3389/fmicb.2017.01490

[26] Michel, Valérie & Martley, Frank. (2001). *Streptococcus thermophilus in Cheddar cheese - Production and fate of galactose.* The Journal of dairy research. 68. 317-25. https://doi.org/10.1017/S0022029901004812

[27] Probiotics.org, (2020), *What is Probiotic S. Thermophilus?*, Retrieved from https://probiotics.org/s-thermophilus/

[28] Zaouche, A., Loukil, C., De Lagausie, P., Peuchmaur, M., Macry, J., Fitoussi, F., Bernasconi, P., Bingen, E., & Cezard, J. P. (2000). *Effects of oral Saccharomyces boulardii on bacterial overgrowth, translocation, and intestinal adaptation after small-bowel resection in rats.* Scandinavian journal of gastroenterology, 35(2), 160–165. https://doi.org/10.1080/003655200750024326

[29] WebMD, (2020), *Saccharomyces Boulardii*, Retrieved from https://www.webmd.com/vitamins/ai/ingredientmono-332/saccharomyces-boulardii

[30] Healthline, (2020), *Probiotics 101: A Simple Beginner's Guide*, Retrieved from https://www.healthline.com/nutrition/probiotics-101

[31] American Dairy Association, (2020), *Greek Yogurt for the Lactose and Gluten Intolerant*, Retrieved from https://www.americandairy.com/news-and-events/dairy-diary/food-and-recipes/greek-yogurt-for-the-lactose-and-gluten-intolerant.stml

[32] Fuller R. (1992) *History and development of probiotics.* In: Probiotics. Springer, https://doi.org/10.1007/978-94-011-2364-8_1

[33] Metchnikoff, E., (1907), *Propagation of Life: Optimistic Studies,* Knickerbocker Press

[34] Guo, R., Chen, L-H., Xing, C., and Liu, T., (2019), *Pain regulation by gut microbiota: molecular mechanisms and therapeutic potential*, British Journal of Anaesthesia, 123(5), 637-654, https://doi.org/10.1016/j.bja.2019.07.026

[35] Davani-Davari, D., Negahdaripour, M., Karimzadeh, I., Seifan, M., Mohkam, M., Masoumi, S. J., Berenjian, A., & Ghasemi, Y. (2019). *Prebiotics: Definition, Types, Sources, Mechanisms, and Clinical Applications.* Foods (Basel, Switzerland), 8(3), 92. https://doi.org/10.3390/foods8030092

7

DIETS

The Good, The Bad, and The Ugly

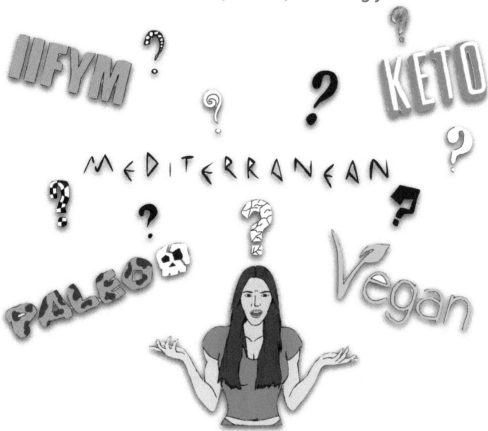

There is no single type of diet that is perfect for everyone on the planet and reduces everyone's risk of disease equally or affects every athlete's performance in the same way. However, that does not stop new diet after new diet popping up and claiming to be a perfect solution for the obesity crisis, cure disease, reduce mortality, extend lifespan, or improve athletic performance. Just follow our guide and don't ask questions is the general message. There are a few underlying healthy themes in most diet plans that can be attributed with the health improvements seen, however, there are some unhealthy habits within some of these diets which are recommended to avoid. Before we delve into these let's look at some of the most popular diets, what is recommended, and how these may or not be beneficial or practical for you.

Mediterranean

Possibly the most widely studied diet in history is the Mediterranean Diet. This diet is based upon following the diet and lifestyle principles of some of the healthiest people in the world, specifically those from the Mediterranean basin. This type of diet has been seen to reduce the risk of several lifestyle diseases such as cardiovascular disease[1], diabetes[2], dementia/Alzheimer's[3], numerous cancers[4] and more[5]. These health benefits are attributed to the anti-inflammatory properties of the foods and practices that comprise a Mediterranean diet. One limitation of such a widely studied diet is the definition of what exactly constitutes a Mediterranean diet due to the Mediterranean covering so many countries and cultures. As a result, different resources may describe this diet a few different ways, often manipulating certain aspects of the diet to meet their individual bias. Therefore, the best resource to use is from the Fundación Dieta Mediterránea[6] for an unbiased description of the Mediterranean diet, which is detailed below:

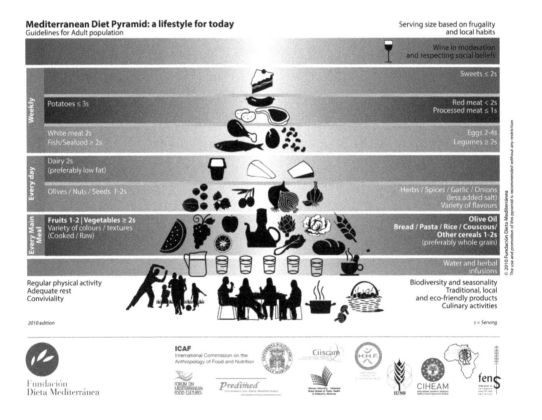

Every Day

- All meals should contain 3 basic elements: cereals (1-2 servings per meal from bread, pasta, rice, couscous etc. preferably wholegrain), vegetables (2+ servings per meal), and fruit (1-2 servings per meal and the default dessert of choice).

- Drink 1.5 – 2 Litres of water/day.
- Moderate amounts of dairy (2 servings per day) with a preference for low-fat dairy or traditional healthier forms such as Greek yoghurt.
- Extra virgin olive oil forms a large part of the Mediterranean diet and should be the primary source of fat used for both cooking and dressing.
- Olives, nuts, and seeds are healthy snack options and another source of good fats.
- Spices, herbs, garlic, and onions are great sources of micronutrients and add flavour and palatability to your meals.
- Alcohol can be consumed at no more than 1 small glass of wine/day for women and 2 glasses/day for men. Alcohol is not a vital part of the Mediterranean diet and can be completely omitted if desired.

Weekly

- Fish and shellfish (2+ servings/week), white meats (2 servings/week), and eggs (2-4 servings/week) are all great sources of protein. A variety of fatty fish is highly recommended including salmon, tuna, mackerel, etc.
- Red meat (less than 2 servings/week) preferably from lean cuts of meat and minimally processed.
- Legumes and pulses (2+ servings/week) are another great source of fibre and plant proteins.
- Potatoes (3 or less servings/week).

Occasionally

- Sweet/sugary foods, heavily processed/refined foods, and unhealthy fats should all be consumed as little as possible with a guide of no more than twice/week. These foods are very calorific and heavily contribute to excess weight gain due to their easy overconsumption.

Cultural/Lifestyle Factors

- In addition to food recommendations, the Mediterranean diet includes lifestyle recommendations that aid in maintaining a healthy balance in your life and encourage healthier eating behaviours and activity levels. These recommendations include: moderate portion sizes, eating with others, cooking, being physically active, and getting adequate rest.

FODMAP

The Low-FODMAP diet is an elimination diet that is often suggested to those experiencing recurring digestive issues like Irritable Bowel Syndrome (IBS)[7]. FODMAP stands for **F**ermentable **O**ligo- **D**i- **M**ono-saccharides

And Polyols, and you may recognise that these are all names for different types of carbohydrates. The FODMAP diet includes a detailed list of foods which are associated with unfavourable symptoms in those with IBS such as bloating, gas, diarrhoea, constipation, and stomach pain[8]. This list is then used to help identify and eliminate IBS symptom trigger foods through careful food tolerance testing and elimination. There are 3 stages to following a Low-FODMAP diet, these are *Restriction*, *Reintroduction*, and *Personalisation*.

Low-FODMAP Foods (Foods to Eat)	High-FODMAP Foods (Foods to Avoid)
Fruits Bananas, blueberries, boysenberries, cantaloupe, cranberries, durian, grapes, grapefruit, honeydew melon, kiwi, lemon, lime, mandarins, oranges, passion fruit, pawpaw, raspberries, rhubarb, rockmelon, strawberries, tangelo	**Fruits** Apples, apricots, avocados, blackberries, cherries, dried fruit, London, lychee, mangos, nashi, nectarines, peaches, pears, persimmon, plums, prunes, tinned fruit in natural juice, watermelon
Vegetables Alfalfa, bamboo shoots, bean shoots, book chop, carrots, choke, chop sum, courgettes, endive, ginger, green beans, lettuce, olives, parsnips, potatoes, pumpkin, red bell peppers, silver beets, spinach, squash, sweet potatoes, tomatoes, turnips, yams	**Vegetables** Artichoke, asparagus, aubergine, beetroot, broccoli, Brussels sprouts, cabbage, cauliflower, fennel, garlic, green bell peppers, leeks, mushrooms, okra, onions, shallots, sweetcorn
Grains Rice, oats, polenta, quinoa, tapioca, some gluten-free products	**Grains** Wheat and rye, couscous, pasta, bread, crackers, cookies
Milk Products Oat milk, rice milk, soy milk, hard cheeses, Brie, Camembert, gelato	**Milk Products** Milk from cows, goats, or sheep, custard, ice cream, yoghurt, soft unripened cheeses such as cottage cheese, mascarpone , ricotta, etc.
Meat Beef, chicken, seafood, pork, eggs (all meat is good basically)	**Legumes & Nuts** Baked beans, chickpeas, kidney beans, lentils, soy beans, pistachios
Other Tofu, sugar (sucrose), glucose, artificial sweeteners not ending in -ol, maple syrup, molasses	**Sweeteners** Corn syrup, honey, fructose, high fructose corn syrup, sorbitol, mannitol, isomalt, maltitol, xylitol

Stage 1 – Restriction

The initial stage of the Low-FODMAP diet involves strict elimination of all High-FODMAP foods for 3 - 8 weeks. How long the initial stage lasts depend on when your digestive symptoms stop. Once you are happy that you are experiencing no more significant digestive symptoms it is time for the next stage.

Stage 2 - Reintroduction

This next stage involves reintroducing individual High-FODMAP foods to first identify which FODMAP foods you can tolerate and then what amount you can tolerate. Each High-FODMAP food needs to be tested alone for 1 - 3 days with the remainder of the diet from the Low-FODMAP food list. This process should be continued until you have tested all the foods from the High-FODMAP list that you are likely to want to consume. Once you have done this its time for the final stage.

Stage 3 - Personalisation

This final stage is now your personalised Low-FODMAP diet, which includes all foods from the original Low-FODMAP list and those identified in stage 2 that you can tolerate well without adverse symptoms.

A major limitation of the FODMAP diet is that IBS is a symptom-driven condition and as such has no one specific treatment[9]. Diet alone may be ineffective at managing the condition and depending on the form of IBS you suffer from medication may also be needed to help manage the symptoms (e.g. constipation sub-type may need regular laxatives whereas the diarrhoea sub-type may require antidiarrheal medication instead). In fact, research has shown that the FODMAP diet is ineffective at managing IBS[10] and more success has been achieved through improving diet diversity and fasting[11], to improve the gut microbiome. Education around triggers for IBS symptoms is also important, as stress can often play a significant role in IBS "flare-ups".

Vegetarian / Vegan

Vegetarian and vegan diets are based upon eliminating animal-derived foods from the diet in varying degrees, for religious, environmental, or personal reasons[12]. Vegetarians do not eat meat or fish but do still consume dairy products and eggs (a.k.a. *Ovo-Lacto Vegetarian*). As a result, vegetarians have good access to several complete protein sources but may lack certain vitamins and minerals such as Vitamin B12 and Iron, as these are best obtained from meat consumption. Some people who eat fish, eggs, and dairy will identify themselves as vegetarian however, this diet is more accurately described as *Pescatarian*.[13] Complete vegetarians (or vegans) do not eat any animal products including all meat, fish, dairy, and eggs[14], and as such are much more limited on quality sources of good bioavailable macro- and micronutrients. Another term often incorrectly used to describe a vegan diet is "plant-based diet". All healthy diets including the

Mediterranean diet described earlier are plant-based, as plants including fruits, vegetables, pulses, and grains etc. form the majority of the diet. A more accurate description for a vegan diet would be a "plant-only diet".

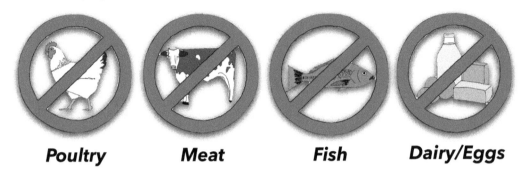

Poultry   **Meat**   **Fish**   **Dairy/Eggs**

Veganism for many is a cultural/lifestyle choice that extends beyond diet and is part of their identity[15]. For this reason, it can be very difficult to highlight the potential deficiencies that can be caused by such a restrictive diet, if not done with careful diet planning and supplementation[16]. Another concern is the potential high usage of meat substitutes by some vegetarians/vegans, which are heavily processed foods. If you are replacing a lean cut of meat, eggs, fish, or dairy, for a ready-made meat substitute then you are making a choice that is worse for your health, not better. There are also a few inflammatory "documentaries" on places like Netflix, that also make claims about meat/dairy/fish/egg consumption on disease risk and performance, based upon cherry-picked studies that are misleading/misrepresent the research. Therefore, if you are considering following or already follow a vegetarian or vegan diet, I strongly suggest having an open-minded discussion with a registered dietician/nutritionist, to ensure you are not missing out on any key nutrients so you can perform at your best in your chosen sport by eating as well-balanced a diet as possible. For example, my wife is vegetarian and even though she is married to a sports nutritionist who cooks for her a varied and healthy diet, she still needs Iron and Vitamin B12 supplementation to prevent low energy levels and fatigue.

Carnivore

The carnivore diet is quite literally the exact opposite of the vegan diet described above. In this case, the recommendation is to consume only animal food sources i.e. meat, fish, eggs, and low-lactose dairy products, based upon the controversial belief that our ancestors ate a predominantly meat and fish only diet[17]. While this is true during times of winter when plant-based foods were scarce, this was quite the opposite during the warmer months in most regions[18]. Much like any diet that requires you to examine the foods you consume more closely, this type of diet can provide several health benefits. However, just like all restriction diets, it comes with potential health concerns such as in this case Vitamin C deficiency and low fibre content. The carnivore diet has no set restrictions on meal frequency, calorie intake, or even serving sizes. As discussed in Chapter 1, diets that are high in protein are beneficial to weight loss due to its satiating effect and its ability to promote muscle protein synthesis. The very high protein consumption from a carnivore diet along with more mindful eating could help to explain why some people find it helpful for weight loss. With limited research into the long-term effects of a carnivore diet on health and performance, I would be reluctant to advocate this type of diet to anyone without a detailed diet plan designed by a registered dietitian/nutritionist.

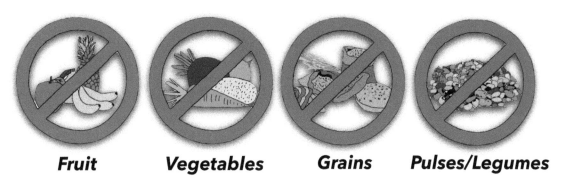

| *Fruit* | *Vegetables* | *Grains* | *Pulses/Legumes* |

Gluten-Free

A gluten-free diet is important to follow for people diagnosed with *Celiac disease*. Celiac disease is an autoimmune disorder where the immune system attacks the intestines in response to eating gluten[19]. This response can cause digestive discomfort and nutrient deficiencies, as foods are not absorbed properly into the body. Celiac disease is hereditary and people with a first-degree relative with the disease (parent, child, or sibling), have a 1 in 10 chance of developing the disease themselves[20]. There is no current treatment option for Celiac disease sufferers, other than life-long adherence to a gluten-free diet.

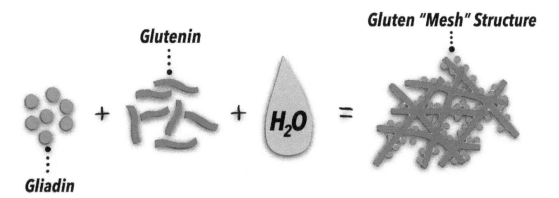

There has been a growing trend in people who do not suffer from Celiac disease following a gluten-free diet for proposed health benefits. However, research published in the British Medical Journal shows that following a gluten-free diet when not diagnosed with Celiac disease can be detrimental to your health[21]. Gluten is a general name for a group of proteins found in wheat that help to bind and maintain the shape of wheat-based foods. As gluten is in a large proportion of complex carbohydrates, eliminating gluten from the diet can lead to losing the health benefits of wholewheat complex carbohydrates on reducing cardiovascular disease. Therefore, unless you have been diagnosed with Celiac disease by a medical professional, it is not advised to follow a gluten-free diet. If you feel you are experiencing digestive issues with wheat-based products first discuss this with a nutritionist to test for Celiac disease, then if you don't have the disease consider increasing the diversity of your diet and reduce your processed foods to improve the diversity of your gut bacteria and your ability to process different food items effectively.

Paleo

The Paleo diet (a.k.a. *The Cave Man Diet*), is based upon pseudoscience theories on what our Palaeolithic ancestors ate before the development of agriculture[22]. This type of diet does not take into consideration several evolutionary processes that have happened to human digestion and makes many assumptions based on little to no evidence or ignoring the evidence all-together. For example, the ability for adults to digest lactose has been traced back to modern-day Turkey, around 8,500 years ago[23], and evidence of the consumption of grains has been found from tools to process the grains and from the tartar on the teeth of Palaeolithic human remains[24]. Some subsets of Paleo dieters also promote eating more raw foods, however, since the discovery of fire our digestive system has decreased in length due to the more efficient extraction of valuable nutrients from cooked foods[25]. Therefore, following a diet that assumes the diet of people that lived as far as 3 million years ago is fundamentally flawed, as the human digestive system, genetics, and food practices have evolved since then.

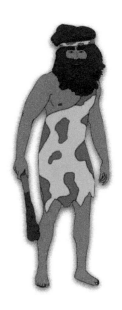

The principles of the Paleo diet are to only consume foods that our Palaeolithic ancestors may have consumed, due to tenuous links made to modern-day agricultural processes and declining human health. The diet involves eating no grains, legumes, dairy, and processed foods while consuming high amounts of fresh foods such as vegetables, fruit, meat, fish, eggs, and tubers (potatoes, turnips, etc.). Despite its deeply flawed pseudoscience background, this type of diet can be somewhat healthy if followed well and focusing more on the reduction of processed foods. However, by eliminating wholegrains the increased risk for cardiovascular disease may be similar to following a gluten-free diet unnecessarily.

Fasting Diets

Intermittent fasting (IF) diets focus less upon the foods consumed and more on the times you are and are not allowed to eat. By restricting caloric intake at specific times, you can help to create a weekly calorie deficit to aid in weight loss, improve insulin resistance, and decrease cardiovascular disease risk. IF has been practised by many religious populations for thousands of years, particularly by Muslims during Ramadan[26]. IF has been heralded as a new magic solution to several health issues including improving cholesterol levels, better blood glucose control, and reducing excess weight. However, when compared to a conventional calorie restriction diet with the same number of total calories consumed on both diet, there is extensive evidence of no significant differences between restricting eating times and eating a conventional meal pattern[27,28,29,30]. Ultimately, the choice of whether to use intermittent fasting to aid with body recomposition comes down to personal preference whereas any other proposed benefits can be achieved by just eating better quality and less quantity of food. Three very popular intermittent fasting diets are *The 5:2 Diet*, *Eat-Stop-Eat*, and *The 16/8 Method*.

The 5:2 Diet

The 5:2 diet involves restricting your calorie consumption to 25% of your caloric needs on any 2 days a week and eating normally the remaining 5 days of the week[31]. This form of intermittent fasting is focused upon weight loss, as this weekly caloric restriction may equal a 3,000 - 3,500 kcal/week deficit (often seen as the equivalent to 1 pound of body fat). The largest drawback to this type of diet is the adherence to a "normal" diet on non-fasting days. If your diet normally consists of unhealthy, high-calorie or heavily processed foods, then your normal daily caloric intake may cause an excess than cancels out the deficit created on fasting days. It may also not improve your health at all as it does not focus on the poor food choices that led to weight gain in the first place.

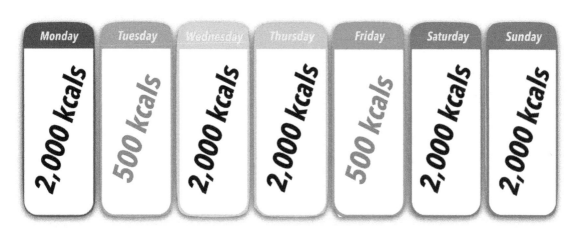

Eat-Stop-Eat

The Eat-Stop-Eat diet involves fasting for 24 to 36 hours on non-consecutive days, 1-2 times a week, then eat normally for the remaining days of the week[32]. For example, having a normal day of eating until 5 pm on Wednesday then not eating again until after 5 pm Thursday. This more extreme length of fasting can be very difficult to adhere to and as such is likely unrealistic for many to be able to adhere to. Performance during such extended fasts may also be notably decreased and as such may not be achievable by athletes with busy training schedules. While most people can skip a meal without experiencing any significant feelings of hunger, particularly on busy days, the mental strength to not eat for an entire 24 – 36 hours is potentially beyond the average person who may already have a poor mental/emotional relationship with food.

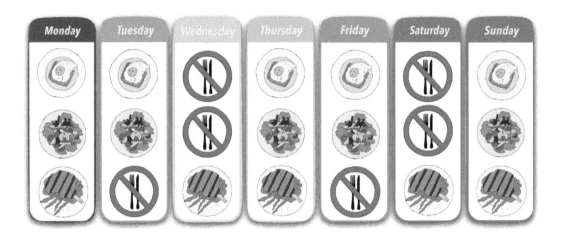

The 16/8 Method

The 16/8 (leangains) method involves simply consuming all of your daily calories within an 8-hour window, followed by a 16 hour fast each day[33]. For example, eating only between 11 am and 7 pm, then fasting from 7 pm until 11 am the next day. The 8-hour eating window you chose is up to your personal preferences on preferred meal times. This is the simplest of the 3-main intermittent fasting methods to follow and the easiest to adhere to over time. Caloric intake varies across days in the 16/8 method, depending upon training or rest days, and training goals (e.g. weight gain, weight loss, or recomposition). Without complete fasting days, the potential hindrance on performance is kept to a minimum. Therefore, if you are considering an intermittent fasting diet, the 16/8 method is the most likely the best option to help improve your health while minimising the effects on your performance.

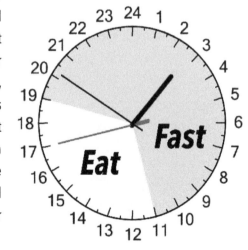

IIFYM (If It Fits Your Macros)

The If It Fits Your Macros (IIFYM) diet originated from an article in the American Dietetic Association newsletter called "all food can fit" in 1996 and relates to discretionary calories left over to meet your caloric needs (approx. 10 - 20% of your TDEE). Around 10 years later online message boards were flooded with questions on the topic, where qualified nutritionists would regularly be asked: "can I eat (insert food) on my diet and still reach my goals?" The nutrition experts started by replying "go ahead if it meets your macronutrient needs then have it". Over time this was shortened to just IIFYM and the more detailed answer has been long forgotten[34]. As a result, the IIFYM concept is now a diet craze with some people feeling it is okay to eat anything they want all the time if it fits their macronutrient needs. This is miles away from the original statement and is not a healthy practice to follow or an effective way of optimising your nutrition for performance.

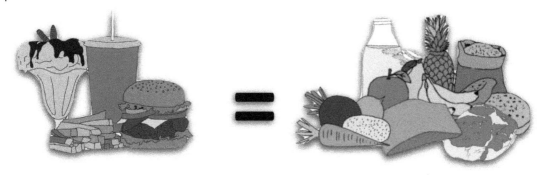

Low-Carb/Keto vs Low-Fat

As the name suggests, a low-carb diet is where the percentage of your diet which is derived from carbohydrates is significantly lower than normal. A "keto" diet (pronounced 'key-toe') gets its name from ketogenesis, a process where your body must create ketone bodies to help ensure enough energy is available for the brain to function normally when not enough carbohydrates are consumed[35]. Ketosis typically occurs when your carbohydrate intake is below 50g/day, whereas the definition of low-carb would be below 130g/day. Some well known low-carb diets include the Atkins diet, the Dukan diet, and even the Paleo diet discussed earlier.

Low-fat diets get their name from the low percentage of total calories which come from dietary fat. In earlier research, dietary fats were labelled as the cause of disease and as such several "low-fat" diets became popular as a way to reduce excess weight and improve health in response to the Seven Countries study by Ancel Keys published in 1970[36]. While low-fat diets can be effective, restricting your intake of dietary fat may lead to nutrient deficiencies and poor mental health due to lost essentials omega-3 Fatty Acids.

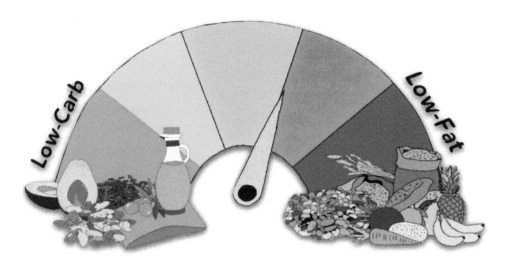

Low-carb and low-fat diets suffer from the same issue in that they try to place the blame of excess weight and poor health on a single macronutrient and do not look at diet quality/quantity, which is the real driver of disease risk. The low-carb movement has been fuelled by a popular theory called the Carbohydrate Insulin Model of Obesity (CIMO), which claims that calories do not matter and that obesity is solely driven by excess dietary carbohydrates causing insulin resistance and gaining of excess fat[37]. Despite proponents of CIMO such as Jason Fung, Gary Taubes, and Robert Lustwig defending this theory regularly, the CIMO has been widely disproven with research showing Calories In vs Calories Out (CICO) remains the foundation of any changes in weight[38] and *there is no significant difference between weight loss and health outcomes from following a low-carb diet vs a low-fat diet when calories and protein intake are kept the same*.

Slimming World® / Weight Watchers®

"Weight loss club" diets have been around for decades and often involve either counting calories or points to achieve weight loss[39,40]. Dieters on these types of diets are typical "yo-yo" dieters, losing large amounts of weight to only regain the weight later. Research shows that diets that focus on solely diet and calorie counting, without a real change in eating and activity behaviour will often fail in this way, with many dieters regaining the weight within 6 months and weighing even heavier 2 years on[41], in part due to the binging behaviour that follows these diet practices. This short-term weight loss can also be explained by the effect long-term obesity has on hormone regulation within the body (i.e. insulin resistance), and the body's desire to create homeostasis as discussed in the energy balance chapter.

While the foods recommended on these diets are mostly good, the demonising of certain foods and small to no encouragement to be more active is where these diets ultimately fail. It is unhealthy to think of foods as "no-no foods" or eliminating them forever as this behaviour is difficult to maintain throughout the entire lifespan without relapse. It is also closed-minded to think that a healthy weight can be maintained through diet alone and to ignore the significant benefits of staying physically active in reducing disease risk. One very positive aspect of weight loss clubs is social support at the weekly meetings. However, this too can come with its pitfalls, as dieters can often perpetuate bad weight loss advice obtained through unreliable sources with no qualified person to advise on these diet myths. For this type of diet to be successful, a dedication toward moving more, learning about the foods you're eating, and remaining sceptical of quick fixes could make this a good option for those who's main focus is sustainable healthy weight loss.

And The Rest...

Meal Replacements (Huel®, SlimFast®, etc.) - the idea of substituting traditional whole-food meals for a liquid food alternative has been around for decades. The quality of meal replacement drinks varies greatly, with newcomer Huel® probably the healthiest of them all to date[42]. Meal replacements are often an effective way to control your calorie intake to stay healthier and/or lose weight. However, *this style of eating does not provide a long-term framework for eating a more nutritious diet due to many people substituting one pre-prepared food item for another and not learning how to create healthier meals for themselves*.

Very Low-Calorie Diets (VLCD) - diets which impose drastic caloric restrictions (i.e. fewer than 800 calories/day), do induce weight loss but also incur a much greater loss in lean mass and greater amounts of metabolic adaptations that reduce your metabolic rate and increase your capacity to regain lost weight[43]. As a result, these diets are extremely poor at achieving long-term weight loss results, can often lead to nutrient deficiencies, and can cause constipation and increased incidence of gallstones[44].

Juice Fasts - A "juice fast" *does not detox your body*. Nor does it have <u>any</u> health benefits. Juice fasts may even be harmful to your health in several ways. Your body has its own detoxification system with your liver and kidneys playing the largest role. No amount of teas, diuretics, or potions will have any positive effect on this system[45].

Alkaline Diet - this diet is based upon reducing the acidity of your body by eating more alkaline foods such as vegetables, nuts, and legumes[46]. However, your diet *does not affect the pH within your blood*. Your body's blood pH levels are predominantly regulated by your lungs and kidneys. Systematic reviews of alkaline diets show urine pH may be altered by alkaline diet but no evidence to support any positive changes to health markers specifically related to alkaline foods[47].

Blue Zones Diet - this diet is based upon trying to eat the same foods as populations in 5 different areas of the world where life expectancy is much higher than normal and the number of centenarians (people who have reached 100 years old) is very high. Together these 5 areas have been described as Blue Zones and include Okinawa - Japan, Sardinia - Italy, Icaria - Greece, Loma Linda - USA, and Nicoya - Costa Rica[48]. However, further research into these populations showed a lack of accurate birth records and high crime rates, suggesting many of these centenarians are falsely claimed, which is evidenced by a drastic decline in centenarian occurrence once more accurate record-keeping was introduced[49].

Low-GI Diet - Primarily aimed at improving blood glucose control in diabetics, or those at a higher risk of developing diabetes (i.e. pre-diabetics)[50]. As discussed in Chapter 1, some foods cause a greater increase in blood sugar levels and can affect the amount of insulin released by the pancreas. However, basing a diet completely on this scoring system does not consider the relative portion sizes of these foods or the health benefits of individual foods that may score more highly. As a result, this is another diet which does not help followers to truly understand the pros and cons of their food choices.

Lactose-Free - Much like the gluten-free diet, avoiding lactose is crucial for people diagnosed with an allergy to lactose. Those with diagnosed lactose-intolerance should try to limit their intake of high lactose foods but may also see improvements in lactose tolerance by improving diet diversity and gut health. If you are not allergic or intolerant to lactose, then there is no need to avoid lactose products[51]. There are also no benefits to avoiding lactose but are some potential health risks due to missing key nutrients such as calcium and very high-quality protein[52].

Blood Type Diet - Your blood type (a.k.a. blood group) is determined by the presence of certain antigens and antibodies within your blood. The most common blood type method used is the ABO system, which indicates the presence of A or B antigens, as well as having neither or both antigens. For example, people with blood group A have A-type antigens and anti-B antibodies[53]. Blood types are essential to know when giving/ receiving blood transfusions, as giving the wrong type blood to someone can be life-threatening. The blood type diet assigns certain diets to individuals based upon their blood type (i.e. type A, B, AB or O), each with a catchy name (i.e. A = cultivator, B = nomad, AB = enigma, O = hunter)[54]. However, the presence of blood typing antigens has no other effect on your health or personality type and basing your diet on this practice is foolhardy. In summary, *there is no scientific evidence to suggest making dietary choices based on your blood type provides any additional benefits and similar results can be obtained by following the diet for any of the 4 blood types*.

Practical Applications

Despite their varying differences, the top healthiest diets do have some recurring themes and practices which can be attributed with the health benefits these diets provide. Therefore, instead of focusing on a named diet, it would be more useful to focus on the recurring themes of these diet types and using the available research, create your own healthy well-balanced diet that takes the best parts of each diet and discards the unnecessary/ unhealthy parts.

When choosing which diet is right for you, you should first consider what you want from your diet. Do you want to improve your health? Do you want to lose weight? Do you want to improve your performance? Can you maintain this type of diet? Do you want a new lifestyle? These seem like obvious questions but many often overlook them and find themselves jumping between diets with mixed levels of success. So before you make your decisions, write down your goals, re-read this chapter, and pick which diet best aligns with your goals and stick to it. Even the best of diets can only work when followed consistently.

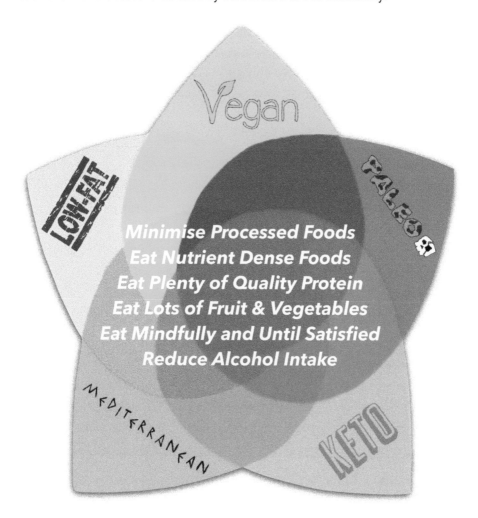

EAT | MOVE | PERFORM **Recommendations**

Using the above common themes between a range of popular diets and drawing upon the other available evidence I have included below my recommendations for a balanced and nutrient-dense diet that will help to keep you healthy and enhance your performance.

1. *Consume 30+ different plants each week.* This includes fruits, vegetables, grains, pulses, legumes, etc. A predominately plant-based diet will provide a host of health benefits to both you and your gut microbiome. While a plant-only diet is not recommended for optimum health and performance, this can be followed for religious or ethical reasons, but requires more careful meal planning.

2. *Eat the rainbow.* This doesn't mean eat lots of Skittles (sorry), it means to choose a wide range of different natural colour foods, as different vitamins, minerals, and phytonutrients are found in higher concentration in different colours of the spectrum.

3. *Consume 80 - 90% minimally processed foods.* Nobody has perfect diet adherence and it's unrealistic to expect this of yourself. Having some sensible levels of flexibility to your diet plan will not only allow you to enjoy social occasions, special events, or even just a relaxed weekend at home guilt-free, it will also keep you on track as no food is on the "no-no" list. Also, if you are eating a well-balanced, nutritious diet 80-90% of the time, the other 10-20% will not undo the health benefits this provides (provided you do not exceed your caloric needs).

4. *When eating meat, the fewer legs the better.* For example, when selecting a meat source choose fish first (no legs), then poultry (2 legs), then everything else (4+ legs).

5. *Consume probiotic dairy products.* Eat a variety of dairy sources including milk, cheese, and yoghurt. Wherever possible this should be from traditional forms such as Greek yoghurt, Skyr, Kefir, etc. which contain beneficial amounts of "good bacteria".

6. *Eat 3 - 6 meals/day.* A minimum of 3 meals/day helps to optimise the number of feeding opportunities you have to take on essentials nutrients, keep you in good health, and fuel performance. Above 6 meals/day is potentially sub-optimal due to the inconvenience this number of eating opportunities would play on your daily life/training schedule and not optimising muscle protein synthesis due to low levels of leucine per meal.

7. *Eat similar sized meals throughout the day.* To optimise how much of the micro- and macronutrients can be released from the food matrix and used by your body you should try to have equal-sized meals throughout the day instead of the typical small breakfast and large dinner scenario.

8. *Drink plenty of water.* Try to have 400 - 500ml of water with your 3 main meals and use a water bottle to rehydrate between meals and when exercising. For a more detailed guide to fluid intake see Chapter 3.

9. *Drink alcohol infrequently and in moderation*. Red wine contains an anti-oxidant called resveratrol which can help reduce your risk of disease. However, this same anti-oxidant is found in fruits so wine consumption isn't essential. To minimise the negative effects of alcohol, select drinks in the following order: wine, clear spirits, dark spirits, spirits with mixers, light colour beer/ale/cider, dark colour beer/ale/cider, stout.

10. *Eat mindfully*. Sit down, ideally with others, chew slowly, do not watch TV or play with your phone. Just focus on what you're eating and take this time to enjoy some downtime.

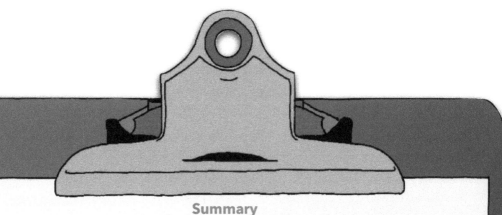

Summary

✓ The Mediterranean diet is the most scientifically supported diet for improving health and reducing disease risk. However, other diets may be just as effective at controlling disease risk if following similar core principles.

✓ A Low-FODMAP diet is often used to help manage IBS symptoms by strategically removing and reintroducing potential trigger foods, however, these types of diets are often ineffective and better results are achieved through increasing diet diversity and managing IBS triggers such as stress.

✓ **Restrictive diets such as Vegan/Vegetarian/Carnivore/Paleo etc. must involve careful diet planning to prevent deficiencies in health and performance** with particular focus placed on increasing diet diversity and possible supplementation for missing nutrients e.g. B12 and Iron for Vegans/Vegetarians.

✓ Fasting diets work by restricting the amount of food you can eat at specific times with the 3 most popular styles being 5:2, Eat-Stop-Eat, or 16/8. **The health benefits of fasting diets come from the caloric deficit they create and they do not have any magical powers**. If you find this form of caloric restriction easier to adhere to than traditional daily caloric restriction then it can be a good option for you for weight management.

✓ You cannot eat whatever you want, whenever you want as long as it fits in with your macronutrient targets (i.e. IIFYM), however, **diet flexibility can aid with adherence.** If take-away food, sweet treats, and other indulgences are limited to only 10-20% of your total caloric intake, then the negative effects of these are minimal and may have little to no effect on your overall goals.

✓ When protein and calories are kept constant, **there is no significant difference between weight loss achieved from a low-carb vs a low-fat diet.** Low-carb diets are not ideal for performance whereas low-fat diets may reduce the amount of healthy fats in your diet and increase disease risk.

✓ "Weight loss club" diets do not teach good long-term skills for eating a balanced diet and often do not include guidance on increasing energy expenditure. As a result, these types of diet often create only short-term, unsustainable weight loss.

✓ **Detox diets are a scam.** Your liver, kidneys, digestive system, and white blood cells will detox your body. Detox diets are more likely to harm your health than improve it.

✓ Most popular diets have recurring themes that can be attributed with the healthy benefits these diets provide. These themes include reducing processed and convenience foods, increasing nutrient-dense foods, eating more mindfully and only until satisfied, and reducing caloric excess from alcohol that reaps the greatest results.

✓ Based upon the available evidence the author recommends consuming 30+ different plants per week, eating a wide range of colours, eating 80-90% minimally processed foods, following a fewer legs the better rule with meat choices, regularly consume probiotic dairy products, eat between 3 and 6 meals per day, eat similar sized meals, stay well-hydrated, drink alcohol only in moderation, and eat mindfully.

REFERENCES

1 Grosso, G., Marventano, S., Yang, J., Micek, A., Pajak, A., Scalfi, L., Galvano, F., & Kales, S. N., (2017) *A comprehensive meta-analysis on evidence of Mediterranean diet and cardiovascular disease: Are individual components equal?*, Critical Reviews in Food Science and Nutrition, 57(15), 3218-3232, https://doi.org/10.1080/10408398.2015.1107021

2 Schwingshackl, L., Missbach, B., König, J., & Hoffmann, G. (2015). *Adherence to a Mediterranean diet and risk of diabetes: A systematic review and meta-analysis*. Public Health Nutrition, 18(7), 1292-1299. https://doi.org/10.1017/S1368980014001542

3 Lourida, I., Soni, M., Thompson-Coon, J., Purandare, N., Lang, I., Ukoumunne, O., & Llewellyn, D. (2013). *Mediterranean Diet, Cognitive Function, and Dementia: A Systematic Review*. Epidemiology, 24(4), 479-489. Retrieved from www.jstor.org/stable/23486687

4 Schwingshackl, L.; Schwedhelm, C.; Galbete, C.; Hoffmann, G., (2017), *Adherence to Mediterranean Diet and Risk of Cancer: An Updated Systematic Review and Meta-Analysis*. Nutrients, 9(10), 1063. https://doi.org/10.3390/nu9101063

5 Dernini, S., Berry, E., Serra-Majem, L., La Vecchia, C., Capone, R., Medina, F., et al., (2017). *Med Diet 4.0: The Mediterranean diet with four sustainable benefits*. Public Health Nutrition, 20(7), 1322-1330. https://doi.org/10.1017/S1368980016003177

6 Fundación Dieta Mediterránea, (2020), *What's the Mediterranean Diet*, Retrieved from https://dietamediterranea.com/en/nutrition/

7 Healthline, (2020), *FODMAP 101: A Detailed Beginner's Guide*, Retrieved from https://www.healthline.com/nutrition/fodmaps-101

8 NHS, (2020), *What is IBS?*, Retrieved from https://www.nhs.uk/conditions/irritable-bowel-syndrome-ibs/

9 Saha L. (2014). *Irritable bowel syndrome: pathogenesis, diagnosis, treatment, and evidence-based medicine*. World journal of gastroenterology, 20(22), 6759–6773. https://doi.org/10.3748/wjg.v20.i22.6759

10 Pimental, M., (2018), *Evidence-Based Management of Irritable Bowel Syndrome With Diarrhea*, American Journal of Managed Care, Retrieved from https://www.ajmc.com/journals/supplement/2018/evidence-based-management-of-ibsd/evidencebased-management-of-irritable-bowel-syndrome-with-diarrhea?p=5

11 Kanazawa, M., Fukudo, S. (2006), *Effects of fasting therapy on irritable bowel syndrome*. International Journal of Behavioural Medicine **13**, 214–220 (2006). https://doi.org/10.1207/s15327558ijbm1303_4

12 Vegetarian Society, (2020), *What is a Vegetarian?*, Retrieved from https://vegsoc.org/info-hub/definition/

13 Healthline, (2020), *What Is a Pescatarian and What Do They Eat?*, Retrieved from https://www.healthline.com/nutrition/pescatarian-diet

14 Vegan Society, (2020), *Definition of Veganism*, Retrieved from https://www.vegansociety.com/go-vegan/definition-veganism

15 Vegan Society, (2020), *Social Identity and Veganism*, Retrieved from https://www.vegansociety.com/about-us/research/research-news/social-identity-and-veganism

16 Pawlak, R., Parrott, S. J., Raj, S., Cullum-Dugan, D., and Lucus, D., (2013), *How prevalent is vitamin B12 deficiency among vegetarians?*, Nutrition Reviews, 71(2), 110–117, https://doi.org/10.1111/nure.12001

17 Healthline, (2020), *All You Need to Know About the Carnivore (All-Meat) Diet*, Retrieved from https://www.healthline.com/nutrition/carnivore-diet/

18 National Geographic Magazine, (2020), *The Evolution of Diet*, Retrieved from https://www.nationalgeographic.com/foodfeatures/evolution-of-diet/

19 Celiac Disease Foundation, (2020), *What is Celiac Disease?*, Retrieved from https://celiac.org/about-celiac-disease/what-is-celiac-disease/

20 Sarno, M., Discepolo, V., Troncone, R., & Auricchio, R. (2015). *Risk factors for celiac disease*. Italian journal of pediatrics, 41, 57. https://doi.org/10.1186/s13052-015-0166-y

21 Lebwohl, B. et al., (2017), *Long term gluten consumption in adults without celiac disease and risk of coronary heart disease: prospective cohort study*, British Medical Journal, 357, J1892, https://doi.org/10.1136/bmj.j1892

22 The Paleo Diet, (2020), *Defining the Paleo Diet*, Retrieved from https://thepaleodiet.com/paleo-101/what-is-paleo

23 Mattar, R., Mazo, D. F. de C., & Carrilho, F. J. (2012). *Lactose intolerance: Diagnosis, genetic, and clinical factors*. Clinical and Experimental Gastroenterology, 5(1), 113-121. http://dx.doi.org/10.2147/CEG.S32368

24 Henry, A. G., Brooks, A. S., and Piperno, D. R., (2011), *Microfossils in calculus demonstrate consumption of plants and cooked foods in Neanderthal diets,* Proceedings of the National Academy of Sciences, 108 (2) 486-491, https://doi.org/10.1073/pnas.1016868108

25 Grand, R. J., Watkins, J. B., and Torti, F. M., (1976), *Development of the Human Gastrointestinal Tract: A Review*, Gastroenterology, 70, 790-810

26 Muslim Hands, (2020), *What is Ramadan?*, Retrieved from https://muslimhands.org.uk/ramadan/what-is-ramadan

27 Seimon, R. V., Roekenes, J. A., Zibellini, J., Zhu, B., Gibson, A. A., Hills, A. P., Wood, R., E., King, N. A., Byrne, N. M., and Sainsbury, A., (2015), *Do intermittent diets provide physiological benefits over continuous diets for weight loss? A systematic review of clinical trials*. Molecular and Cellular Endocrinology, 15, 418, Pt 2, 155-172, https://doi.org/10.1016/j.mce.2015.09.014

28 Headland, M., Clifton, P. M., Carter, S., & Keogh, J. B. (2016). *Weight-Loss Outcomes: A Systematic Review and Meta-Analysis of Intermittent Energy Restriction Trials Lasting a Minimum of 6 Months*. Nutrients, 8(6), 354, https://doi.org/10.3390/nu8060354

29 Harris, L., Hamilton, S., Azevedo, L. B., Olajide, J., De Brún, C., Waller, G., Whittaker, V., Sharp, T., Lean, M., Hankey, C., & Ells, L. (2018). *Intermittent fasting interventions for treatment of overweight and obesity in adults: a systematic review and meta-analysis*. JBI database of systematic reviews and implementation reports, 16(2), 507–547. https://doi.org/10.11124/JBISRIR-2016-003248

30 Cioffi, I., Evangelista, A., Ponzo, V., Ciccone, G., Soldati, L., Santarpia, L., Contaldo, F., Pasanisi, F., Ghigo, E., & Bo, S. (2018). *Intermittent versus continuous energy restriction on weight loss and cardiometabolic outcomes: a systematic review and meta-analysis of randomized controlled trials*. Journal of translational medicine, 16(1), 371. https://doi.org/10.1186/s12967-018-1748-4

31 Mosley, M., (2014), *The Fasting Diet*, Short Books Ltd.

32 Pilon, B., (2007), *Eat Stop Eat*, Self Published

33 Leangains, (2020), *The Leangains Guide*, Retrieved from https://leangains.com/the-leangains-guide/

34 Aragon, A., (2019), *IIFYM History Lesson*, Retrieved from https://www.instagram.com/p/B088PtJBJMI/?igshid=qfcdo4uevd70

35 Healthline, (2020), *Checking Ketone Levels*, Retrieved from https://www.healthline.com/health/type-2-diabetes/facts-ketones#prevention

36 Keys A., (1970), *Coronary heart disease in seven countries*. Circulation. 41(S1):118-139.

37 Ludwig, D. S., & Ebbeling, C. B. (2018). *The Carbohydrate-Insulin Model of Obesity: Beyond "Calories In, Calories Out"*. JAMA internal medicine, 178(8), 1098–1103. https://doi.org/10.1001/jamainternmed.2018.2933

38 Gardner, C. D., Trepanowski. J. F., Del Gobbo, L. C., Hauser, M. E., Rigdon, J., Ioannidis, J., Desai, M., & King, A. C. (2018). *Effect of Low-Fat vs Low-Carbohydrate Diet on 12-Month Weight Loss in Overweight Adults and the Association With Genotype Pattern or Insulin Secretion*: The DIETFITS Randomized Clinical Trial. JAMA, 319(7), 667–679. https://doi.org/10.1001/jama.2018.0245

39 Slimming World, (2020), *How does it work?*, Retrieved from https://www.slimmingworld.co.uk/how-it-works

40 Weight Watchers, (2020), *How it WW work?*, Retrieved from https://www.weightwatchers.com/uk/how-it-works

[41] Hall, K. D., & Kahan, S. (2018). *Maintenance of Lost Weight and Long-Term Management of Obesity*. The Medical clinics of North America, *102*(1), 183–197. https://doi.org/10.1016/j.mcna.2017.08.012

[42] Huel, (2020), *About Us*, Retrieved from https://huel.com/pages/about-us

[43] Dulloo, A. G., Jacquet, J., & Montani, J. P. (2012). *How dieting makes some fatter: from a perspective of human body composition autoregulation*. The Proceedings of the Nutrition Society, *71*(3), 379–389. https://doi.org/10.1017/S0029665112000225

[44] Rolland, C., Mavroeidi, A., Johnston, K. L., & Broom, J. (2013). The effect of very low-calorie diets on renal and hepatic outcomes: a systematic review. *Diabetes, metabolic syndrome and obesity : targets and therapy, 6*, 393–401. https://doi.org/10.2147/DMSO.S51151

[45] Klein, A.V. & Kiat, H. (2015), *Detox diets for toxin elimination and weight management: a critical review of the evidence*. Journal of Human Nutrition and Dietetics. 28, 675– 686, https://doi.org/10.1111/jhn.12286

[46] Healthline, (2020), *The Alkaline Diet: An Evidence-Based Review*, Retrieved from https://www.healthline.com/nutrition/the-alkaline-diet-myth

[47] Remer, T., & Manz, F. (1995). *Potential renal acid load of foods and its influence on urine pH*. Journal of the American Dietetic Association, *95*(7), 791–797. https://doi.org/10.1016/S0002-8223(95)00219-7

[48] Buettner, D., (2009), *The Blue Zones*, National Geographic

[49] Newman, S. J., (2019), *Supercentenarians and the oldest-old are concentrated into regions with no birth certificates and short lifespans*, Retrieved from https://doi.org/10.1101/704080

[50] Mayo Clinic, (2020), *Glycemic Index Diet: What's behind the claims,* Retrieved from https://www.mayoclinic.org/healthy-lifestyle/nutrition-and-healthy-eating/in-depth/glycemic-index-diet/art-20048478

[51] Healthline, (2020), *Is Dairy Bad for You, or Good? The Milky, Cheesy Truth*, Retrieved from https://www.healthline.com/nutrition/is-dairy-bad-or-good

[52] Hoffman, J. R., & Falvo, M. J. (2004). *Protein - Which is Best?*. Journal of sports science & medicine, *3*(3), 118–130.

[53] Encyclopaedia Britannica, (2020), *ABO blood group system*, Retrieved from https://www.britannica.com/science/ABO-blood-group-system

[54] D'Adamo, P., (2017), *Eat Right 4 Your Type*, Berkley

8

SUPPLEMENTS

Useful benefits or a big waste of money?

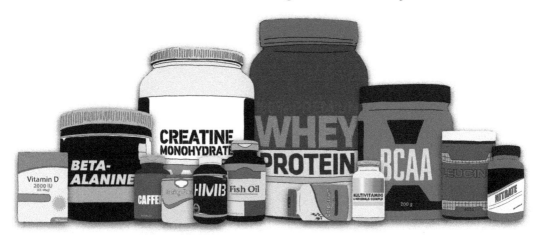

Dietary supplements are substances that can be taken to improve health and/or athletic performance. The use of supplements for general health may be an effective way to meet potential deficiencies created by underlying medical conditions or restrictive diet practices (e.g. Vitamin C for carnivore dieters). Supplements for performance focus on substances that when taken provide an ergogenic aid (e.g. taking creatine for short duration exercise performance). This chapter is far from an exhaustive review of all the available supplements but instead has focused on some of the most popular, legal, and well-researched supplements to date. To help guide you, this chapter is divided into supplements that have strong evidence for their potential use, some evidence, and weak/no evidence.

Strong Evidence

Beta-Alanine (a.k.a. β-alanine)

Beta-alanine is a modified version of the amino acid alanine and has been shown to improve muscular endurance. This translates as being able to perform 1 - 2 extra reps when training in the 8 - 15 rep range, or improvements in moderate- to high-intensity cardiovascular exercise (e.g. rowing or sprinting)[1]. Beta-alanine is converted in the body to carnosine, which buffers acid in the muscles lowering pH. This is particularly beneficial to attenuate exercise-induced pH increases from lactic acid production and diet-induced pH increases, which may occur on very low-carb (keto) diets[2].

Dosage: 2 - 5 g.

Timing: Often found in pre-workout formulas but has no specific timing requirements.

Side Effects: Beta-alanine supplements can sometimes cause a tingling sensation called paresthesia. This is a harmless side effect but may be avoided by taking smaller (0.8 - 1.0 g) doses several times/day or using a time-release formulation.

Best For: Exercise bouts lasting 60 - 240 seconds such as weightlifting or moderate to vigorous-intensity cardiovascular exercise.

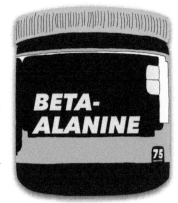

Caffeine

Caffeine is found naturally in coffee beans and tea but can also be synthesised to make supplements. *Caffeine is a powerful stimulant that can be used to enhance both strength and endurance performance*[3]. Caffeine is a nootropic that sensitises neurones and provides mental stimulation by antagonising adenosine receptors. Regular caffeine consumption is associated with a reduced risk of cardiovascular disease, Alzheimer's, and liver cancer. However, habitual caffeine use can lead to increased tolerance and its effects becoming diminished[4]. Taking a month-long break from regular caffeine use may help to reduce tolerance/increase sensitivity.

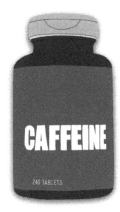

Dosage: Approx. 3 - 6 mg/kg. Tailor to individual by starting with the minimal effective dose and increasing if/when tolerance increases. Greater effect seen when taken in anhydrous supplements than from coffee.

Timing: 20 - 30 minutes before exercise. Avoid caffeine within 4 hours of bedtime to avoid sleep disturbances.

Side Effects: Excess caffeine consumption can cause sleep disturbances, heart arrhythmias, and even death.

Best For: Increased power output (both weightlifting and cycling) as well as and anaerobic running capacity.

Creatine

Creatine is the most widely studied sports supplement with thousands of research papers detailing its benefits in both health and performance. *Creatine is a compound that is formed in the liver, kidneys, and pancreas from amino acids and is used to replenish ATP through the Phosphocreatine System* (See Chapter 1). Creatine is found naturally in meat and fish, however, the amount found in food is often not sufficient to provide an ergogenic effect. In sport, creatine is primarily used to increase work capacity for exercises lastly less than 30 seconds in length such as weightlifting, sprinting, or any short bursts of maximum effort.

Therefore, it can be particularly useful for gaining lean muscle mass and increasing strength[5]. Recent studies have shown potential benefits of creatine supplementation on cognitive performance and brain health although this research is still somewhat in its infancy. Creatine levels are significantly lower in vegetarians, vegans, and the elderly and as such these populations can benefit greatly from its use[6].

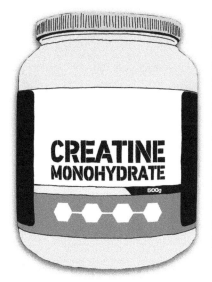

Dosage: Best used with a loading protocol of 0.3 g/kg/day for 5 -7 days then 0.03 g/kg/day to maintain saturation. A simplified guide is 20g per day for 1 week followed by 2-3 g per day to maintain or 2-3 g per day with no loading protocol (although saturation will take longer and results may be lower).

Timing: Creatine can be taken at any time in the day that is convenient to meet the strategies detailed above. It is often included in pre-workout supplements.

Side Effects: Stomach cramping if taken without sufficient water or nausea and diarrhoea if too large of doses taken at once.

Best For: Increasing power output and muscular hypertrophy.

Fish Oils

Fish oils refers to the Omega-3 fatty acids EPA and DHA discussed in Chapter 2. While these fatty acids can be synthesised in small amounts from ALA within your body, it is much more readily available from oily fish[7]. For those who dislike fish or simply do not consume it often enough, *fish oil supplements are a great way to help ensure sufficient amounts of EPA & DHA are achieved*.

Dosage: 250 - 1,000 mg per day of combined EPA & DHA.

Timing: Advised to spread the dosage out across the day to avoid potential fishy tasting burps.

Side Effects: No significant side effects other than the above mentioned fishy burps.

Best For: Depression and reducing triglyceride levels.

Protein

Protein supplements are an effective way to help you reach your recommended intake of protein when struggling to do so from diet alone. *Protein supplements can be a more convenient way to reach your daily protein requirements*. However, if you are meeting your daily recommended intake of protein from your diet, protein supplements will not add any additional ergogenic benefits. For detailed information on recommended protein intake and timing see Chapters 2 and 4 respectively.

Sodium Bicarbonate

Sodium bicarbonate (a.k.a. baking soda or baking powder) acts as a buffering agent for acidity within your body[8]. *Sodium Bicarbonate can help to reduce the "burning' sensation felt within the muscles during intense exercise and subsequently increase work capacity*.

Dosage: Approx. 200 - 300 mg/kg although up to 500 mg/kg may be more effective.

Timing: 60 - 90 minutes before exercise. For longer duration exercise 45 - 60 minutes before exercise may be better.

Side Effects: Possible gastric distress including stomach and nausea leading to diarrhoea and flatulence if taken too quickly or with higher doses. Consuming smaller doses may help reduce potential side effects.

Best For: Increased aerobic exercise work capacity.

Vitamin D

During the warmer months (i.e. April - October in the Northern Hemisphere), the majority of Vitamin D is best obtained from UVB sunlight (UV index of 3 or higher) by exposing a large area of skin to the sun for 30 minutes per day[9]. However, *with the majority of people now working indoors during peak sunlight hours and potential bad weather, there is a need for potential Vitamin D supplementation* to ensure sufficient amounts are obtained to remain in good health.

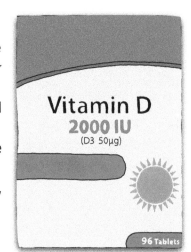

Dosage: For effective dosing supplements are much higher than the RDA for Vitamin D with 1,000 - 2,000 IU/day doses and with an upper limit of 4,000 IU/day.

Timing: Best taken with meals that include 3 - 5 grams of fat to aid absorption.

Side Effects: Virtually none but possible Hypervitaminosis D in rare cases with extreme doses over 10,000 IU/day.

Best For: Reduced cardiovascular disease, multiple sclerosis, fall risk, asthma attacks, fracture risk, and thyroid issues.

Some Evidence

Branched Chain Amino Acids (BCAAs)

As discussed in Chapter 2, BCAAs include the essential amino acids leucine, isoleucine, and valine and play a significant role in muscular hypertrophy (i.e. muscle growth). *BCAAs can be derived from diet alone and supplemental use does not deliver any performance benefits over dietary sources*. However, there is a moderate benefit from BCAA supplementation for those not meeting their protein requirements from their diet.[10]

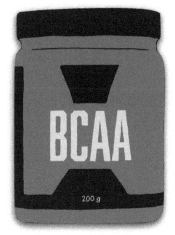

Dosage: A combined dose of 20g with a balanced ratio of leucine, isoleucine, and valine.

Timing: To be taken throughout the day along with dietary protein.

Side Effects: No known side effects.

Best For: Muscle growth and strength when dietary protein is insufficient to meet daily protein recommendations.

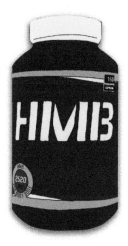

β-Hydroxy β-Methylbutyric Acid (HMB)

HMB is an active metabolite of leucine that reduces muscle protein breakdown. *HMB has anti-catabolic effects which attenuates muscle protein breakdown*. HMB is more effective than leucine at attenuating muscle protein breakdown but less effective on muscle protein synthesis. Therefore, the use of HMB may be beneficial in aiding to meeting leucine/protein requirements[11].

Dosage: 1 -3 g/daily.

Timing: 30 - 45 minutes before a workout.

Side Effects: No known side effects.

Best For: Reducing muscle protein breakdown/muscle damage.

Colostrum

Colostrum is the pre-milk fluid secreted by mammals that have recently given birth. This unique fluid has *similar benefits to whey protein on MPS and also aids immune and digestive health*[12].

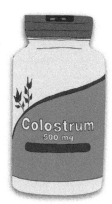

Dosage: 20 - 60 g or 400 - 3,500 mg when used for digestive health.

Timing: Nothing specific.

Side Effects: None known.

Best For: Muscle protein synthesis, immune and digestive health.

Leucine

As noted in Chapter 2, leucine is pivotal in boosting MPS and is one of the 3 BCAAs. *Leucine taking in isolation may be a cheaper alternative to BCAA supplements but may not be as effective*. Leucine alone is also less effective than whole protein supplements with optimised leucine content such as whey and casein.

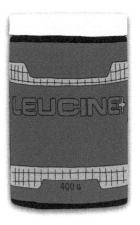

Dosage: 2,000 - 5,000 mg in a fasted state[13].
Timing: Taken with low protein quality meals.
Side Effects: None known.
Best For: Optimising MPS in poor-quality protein diets where animal source proteins may not be an option.

Multi-Vitamins

Multi-vitamins can be an effective way to meet any of the missing micronutrients from a healthy and varied diet. However, *multi-vitamins do not offer any additional benefits to health and/or performance if*

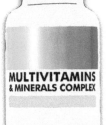

all essential nutrients are found in your diet[14]. As noted before, you may like to use a multi-vitamin as a kind of "insurance policy" but never as a substitute for a good diet.

Dosage: Varies depending on content and requirements.
Timing: Usually once per day with food.
Side Effects: Potential for hypervitaminosis but uncommon if taking the recommended dose.
Best For: Individuals on a restrictive diet such as vegetarian/vegans, carnivore, paleo, gluten-free or similar. Best to discuss with your GP or nutritionist for a more detailed recommendation.

Nitrate

Nitrate rich foods include leafy greens and root vegetables (i.e. spinach, rocket, celery, beetroot etc.), although beetroot juice is the most commonly used for supplementation. *Nitrates can aid performance by increasing nitric oxygen synthase which stimulates the dilation of the blood vessels*. This, in turn, increases blood flow, oxygen uptake and endurance capacity as well as cardiovascular health[15].

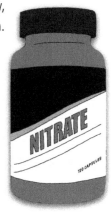

Dosage: 0.1 - 0.2 mmol/kg (or 6.4 - 12.8 mg/kg) or beetroot juice.
Timing: Within 8 hours before exercise.
Side Effects: None known.
Best For: Improving aerobic exercise capacity (particularly running), lowering blood pressure and subsequently cardiovascular disease risk.

Weak/No Evidence

Conjugated Linoleic Acid (CLA)

CLA are fatty acids that are sold as "fat burners" as they affect a cell signal pathways called Peroxisome proliferator-activated receptors (PPARs). However, *the effect of CLA on PPARs is insufficient to have any noticeable effect on fat loss*. CLA also has claims on aiding inflammation, and glucose/lipid metabolism however, there is no reliable evidence to support these claims and the overall effect size of these studies does not support these claims[16]. In summary, the only thing CLA burns is your money.

Green Tea Extract

Green tea extract is another supplement with fat burner claims but with very little evidence to back it up[17]. Green tea contains polyphenols which may offer health benefits. However, *research to date shows limited evidence to support the use of green tea for fat loss or improvements in key health markers*. Save your money and focus more on energy balance. For the proposed benefits enjoy a cup of green tea or a cup of coffee instead.

Zinc, Magnesium Aspartate, & Vitamin B6 (ZMA)

Testosterone is the male growth hormone which has a significant impact on muscle mass and strength. The use of anabolic agents including steroids and growth hormones is widespread in bodybuilding and these agents 100% increase the amount of lean muscle mass you can accumulate. Testosterone boosters, on the other hand, are dietary supplements which claim to naturally boost your testosterone levels through dietary intervention. The most popular testosterone booster is called ZMA, which is a combination of aspartate with key vitamins and minerals. Aspartate is claimed to increase testosterone level but is too low of a dose in ZMA supplements to significantly affect testosterone levels. In fact, the most compelling study to date showing a significant ergogenic benefit for taking ZMA supplements was published by the creators of ZMA[18], coincidence? Probably not. *A review of different methods on boosting testosterone levels shows that supplements like ZMA have a similar benefit to watching an exciting action movie*. Therefore, forget the pills and pop on one of the Rocky movies or Gladiator pre-workout instead.

Practical Applications

Before you decide to start using dietary supplements you must first ensure that you have followed the food first approach and optimised your diet. I would then recommend following the 4 steps plan (see below) proposed by Graham Close PhD, a respected sports nutritionist and professor of human physiology when making your decisions about whether or not using a particular supplement is the right thing for you[19].

1. Do You Need It

The supplement industry is a multi-billion dollar business worldwide with an invested interest in you buying their latest training aid. But do you really need it? If you are an average Joe looking to stay healthy then at best you may need a multi-vitamin but if you are more regularly active or an athlete then there is more to consider. When assessing your need for supplementation you should first see if you can get the active ingredient from your food in sufficient amounts to have an ergogenic benefit because if you can then it makes sense to do so. Next, do your research - supplement companies and "influencers" will cherry-pick research to get you to buy their product. Try to remain sceptical, dig a little deeper, and where possible try to look at the meta-analyses of available data. If there is limited to no data, give it a miss. Finally, context is key. The effect of a supplement in one sport or training style may not translate to your sport or training. Make sure you only take supplements that have been proven to benefit your goals specifically. A great resource to check for yourself is **www.examine.com** which is a free service that shows you the evidence behind your supplements and their claims.

2. What Are The Pros & Cons?

As with most decisions in life weighing up the pros and cons of taking an action is always a good idea. To start with, always be wary of supplement claims. If it seems to good to be true then it probably is. While some of these products may deliver the results they claim, they can often be at the expense of your health or even your life. Do you know what's in it? Check through the ingredients list and google anything you don't recognise. If you're an athlete, make sure none of the listed ingredients are on the World Anti-Doping Agency (WADA) banned list. Is the concentration of the active ingredient enough to do what it says. For example, ZMA supplements contain not enough aspartate to have a significant effect on serum testosterone levels. For athletes, the most effective way to be safe and not waste your money is to not take any supplements at all. However, this may mean losing some significant performance benefits. Therefore, the next best thing is to only use products that have been proven to enhance performance and follow strict batch control tests which we'll cover next.

3. Finding a Safe/Trusted Product

In 2014, 10.5% of 152 available supplements in the UK tested positive for banned substances on the World Anti-Doping Violations List. Furthermore, in 2012 44% of UK anti-doping failed tests were due to prohibited substances within over-the-counter supplements.

Supplement Use Flow-Chart

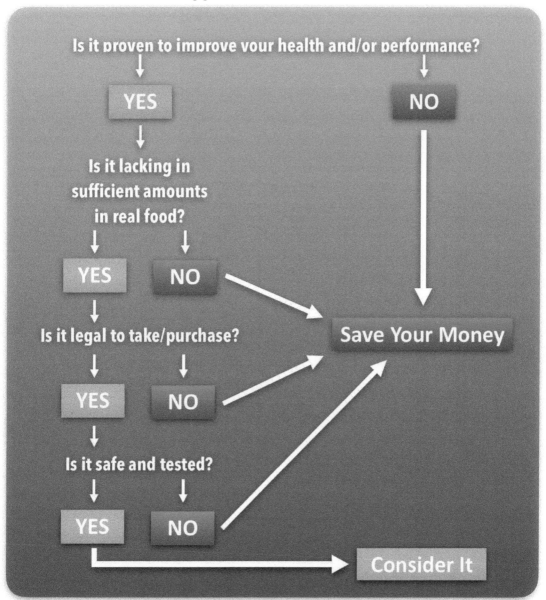

If you are an athlete, in regular competition it is your responsibility to know what constitutes a doping violation as ignorance is not deemed an acceptable excuse. For non-athletes, the main concern is with your health and not taking supplements that may be contaminated with substances that could harm your health. Banned/harmful substances may be within your supplements due to poor manufacturing processes, contaminated raw ingredients, or deliberate spiking. To clarify, deliberate spiking may not be someone slipping it into your drink while you're not looking, rather it is the deliberate adding of a known performance-enhancing drug to increase the effects of the supplement. Recent examples of this include methamphetamines found within some pre-workouts, now that really will get you pumped up and it did so the pre-workout in question flew off the shelves. Another great resource is the Informed-Sport service (**www.informed-sport.com**), which certifies products that have been manufactured in a way that adheres to the WADA regulations for each specific batch. However, be careful of some unscrupulous companies using the informed sport logo illegally and check the informed sport website to double-check before purchase.

When it comes to putting things into your body you cannot be too careful. Plus, the most effective supplements can all be purchased cheaply from reputable companies and/or found in sufficient amounts in food. Therefore, before buying any supplements online or in stores, do some research into the ingredients and check with Informed Sport (if applicable) to keep you safe and healthy.

4. Non-Responders

Let's say you've followed all the above advice and have been using a supplement for several months and training hard but you haven't noticed any training benefits or changes in your blood results. Should you keep taking it? My answer would be no! In every piece of research, there are always "non-responders", those few individuals who do not respond in the way we would expect to supplements or an exercise stimulus. If you've been doing everything right but noticing no improvements then maybe its time to cut your losses and save your money.

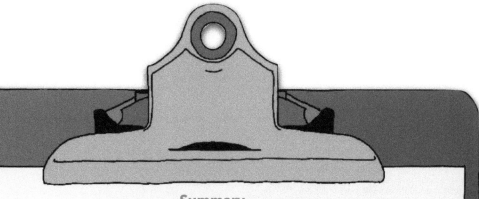

Summary

✓ **Supplements are a non-essential but potentially beneficial addition to your nutrition plan**.

✓ Popular supplements with strong evidence to support their use include **Beta-Alanine**, **Caffeine**, **Creatine**, **Fish Oils**, **Protein**, **Sodium Bicarbonate**, and **Vitamin D**.

✓ Beta-Alanine and Sodium Bicarbonate can aid muscular endurance.

✓ Caffeine can aid both strength and endurance performance.

✓ Fish Oils and Vitamin D are helpful to ensure you meet your RDA of these key nutrients.

✓ Popular supplements with some evidence to support their use include **BCAAs**, **HMB**, **Colostrum**, **Leucine**, **Multi-Vitamins**, and **Nitrate**.

✓ Popular supplements with weak to no evidence to support their use include **CLA**, **Green Tea Extract**, and Testosterone Boosters (e.g. **ZMA**).

✓ Before deciding to use any supplements you should **consider whether you need it**, **what are the pros and cons of use**, **is the supplement safe and tested**, and **consider that some are non-responders**.

✓ The website **Examine.com** is a useful resource to find evidence-based information about most popular supplements.

✓ **Be careful of where you buy your supplements as many supplements contain substances that may be detrimental to your health** or cause a failed rugs test if competing as an athlete.

✓ To help find trusted products the website **Informed-Sport.com** is a useful resource.

✓ To fully understand what counts as a doping violation check out the WADA regulations. Not knowing what constitutes a doping violation is not an acceptable excuse and could see you banned from your sport for up to 4 years.

REFERENCES

[1] Hobson RM, Saunders B, Ball G, Harris RC, Sale C. (2012), *Effects of β-alanine supplementation on exercise performance: a meta-analysis*. Amino Acids. 43(1), 25-37. https://doi.org/10.1007/s00726-011-1200-z

[2] Examine.com, (2020), *Beta-Alanine*, Retrieved from https://examine.com/supplements/beta-alanine/

[3] Doherty, M., & Smith, P. M. (2004). *Effects of Caffeine Ingestion on Exercise Testing: A Meta-Analysis*, International Journal of Sport Nutrition and Exercise Metabolism, 14(6), 626-646, https://doi.org/10.1123/ijsnem.14.6.626

[4] Examine.com, (2020), *Caffeine*, Retrieved from https://examine.com/supplements/caffeine/

[5] Branch, J. (2003). *Effect of Creatine Supplementation on Body Composition and Performance: A Meta-analysis*, International Journal of Sport Nutrition and Exercise Metabolism, 13(2), 198-226, https://doi.org/10.1123/ijsnem.13.2.198

[6] Examine.com, (2020), *Creatine*, Retrieved from https://examine.com/supplements/creatine/

[7] Examine.com, (2020), *Fish* Oils, Retrieved from https://examine.com/supplements/fish-oil/

[8] Examine.com, (2020), *Sodium Bicarbonate*, Retrieved from https://examine.com/supplements/sodium-bicarbonate/

[9] Examine.com, (2020), *Vitamin D*, Retrieved from https://examine.com/supplements/vitamin-d/

[10] Examine.com, (2020), **Branched Chain Amino Acids**, Retrieved from https://examine.com/supplements/branched-chain-amino-acids/

[11] Examine.com, (2020), *Summary of HMB*, Retrieved from https://examine.com/supplements/hmb/

[12] Examine.com, (2020), *Summary of Colostrum*, Retrieved from https://examine.com/supplements/colostrum/

[13] Examine.com, (2020), *Summary of Leucine*, Retrieved from https://examine.com/supplements/leucine/

[14] Macpherson, H., Pipingas, A., and Pase, M. P., (2013), *Multivitamin-multimineral supplementation and mortality: a meta-analysis of randomized controlled trials*, The American Journal of Clinical Nutrition, 97(2), 437–444, https://doi.org/10.3945/ajcn.112.049304

[15] Examine.com, (2020), *Summary of Nitrate*, Retrieved from https://examine.com/supplements/nitrate/

[16] Examine.com, (2020), *Summary of Conjugated Linoleic Acid*, Retrieved from https://examine.com/supplements/conjugated-linoleic-acid/

[17] Hursel, R., Viechtbauer, W. & Westerterp-Plantenga, M. (2009), *The effects of green tea on weight loss and weight maintenance: a meta-analysis*. International Journal of Obesity, **33,** 956–961. https://doi.org/10.1038/ijo.2009.135

[18] Brilla, L. R., & Conte, V., (2000), *Effects of a Novel Zinc-Magnesium Formulation on Hormones and Strength*, Journal of Exercise Physiology, 3 (4), Retrieved from http://wikigimnasio.com/wp-content/uploads/Effects-of-a-Novel-Zinc-Magnesium-Formulation-on-Hormones-and-Strength.pdf

[19] Close, G., (2018), *Supplements and the Athlete*, UK Strength and Conditioning Association Annual Conference

APPENDIX

Below is a step-by-step plan for you to create your personalised nutrition plan, utilising all the information you have learned so far. I have divided the step-by-step guide into General Health guidelines and Performance guidelines as well as a generic example diet plan for 2,000 calorie typical week.

General Health Guidelines

Step 1 - Calculate your caloric needs
Calculate your BMR using either the Müller et al. or Harris-Benedict equation and multiply this number by the relevant activity factor. Your resulting TDEE will usually be within 200-300 calories of these calculations so use a little trial and error to determine the right amount for you. If you are trying to lose fat then you need to eat below your TDEE, if you are trying to gain muscle then eat 250-500 calories above your TDEE. For maintenance, just eat your TDEE, monitor your weight, and make adjustments if necessary.

Calculate your protein, fat, and carbohydrate requirements - Step 2
Calculate your protein requirements based upon your goals and type of physical activity you are engaging in. For example, consume 1.6 – 2.2g/kg/day for weight loss. Multiple you total protein intake in grams by 4 to calculate total daily calories from protein and substrate this from your target TDEE. For general health, the remaining calories can come from any ratio of fat and carbohydrates but try to avoid the extreme ends of the spectrum. A good rule of thumb for most people is to consume 50% of your total calories from carbohydrates and less than 35% from fat (<11% saturated fats, 6.5% from polyunsaturated fats, 13% monounsaturated fats).

Step 3 – Optimise your nutrient intake and prevent deficiencies
To help ensure optimum levels of micronutrients within your diet you should aim to consume a wide variety of foods, aiming for 30+ different plant foods per week and a wide range of colours. This greater level of diversity will also help to improve your gut microbiome and enhance the bioavailability of your diet. If you chose to follow a restriction diet (i.e. vegan, gluten-free, paleo, etc.) it is important to consider the need to supplement key micronutrients, which may not be obtained in sufficient amounts to keep you in good health. To aid bioavailability, try to include some of the food combinations listed in Chapter 5.

Calculate hydration needs around your meals and exercise - Step 4

Basic population guidance suggests men should consume 2.0 - 2.5 litres of fluid per day and women 1.5 - 2.0 litres of fluid per day. A simple strategy to achieve this is to have a large 400-500 ml glass of water with each of your 3 main meals and then sip from a drinks bottle between meals to meet the remaining requirements. I recommended using a clear water bottle as this can act as a useful visual feedback to drink more often when kept nearby.

Step 5 - Include some flexibility and plan for special events

You don't need perfect diet adherence to be happy and healthy. Following a well-balanced, nutrient-dense diet that is 80 - 90% of your total caloric intake allows you to enjoy less healthier options the remaining 10 - 20% of your caloric intake. However, if you know you will exceed you caloric intake goals due to a special occasion (e.g. birthday party, wedding, night out with friends, etc.), or you know you are more likely to overindulge on certain days of the week (e.g. Saturday and Sunday), then planning for this ahead of time can keep you on track. For example, take your TDEE and increase this by however much you feel you may over-consume on a set day. Then divide how much extra you are consuming on that day by the remaining other days in the week and decrease your TDEE for each of those days by this amount. Remember, as long as your weekly energy intake (i.e. your TDEE x7) is not exceeded you will not gain excess fat.

Performance Guidelines

Calculate your caloric needs - Step 1

Calculate your BMR using either the Müller et al. or Harris-Benedict equation and multiply this number by the relevant activity factor. Your resulting TDEE will usually be within 200-300 calories of these calculations so use a little trial and error to determine the right amount for you. If you are trying to lose fat to 'make weight' then you need to eat below your TDEE. Aim to lose no more than 1% of your total bodyweight per week to help maintain as much lean muscle mass as possible. Utilising an uneven daily caloric restriction to allow for strategic re-feeding may also maintain more lean muscle mass during a caloric deficit. If you are trying to gain lean muscle mass then eat 250-500 calories above your TDEE. Monitor this amount and adjust as necessary if you start to gain too much fat. For general performance just meet your TDEE.

Step 2 - Calculate your protein, fat, and carbohydrate requirements

Calculate your protein requirements based upon your goals and type of physical activity you are engaging in. For example, consume 1.6 – 2.2g/kg/day for strength and power-based sports. Next, calculate your carbohydrate requirements based on your training needs. Concert your protein and carbohydrate intake in grams in calories (i.e. 4 calories/gram for both protein and carbs) and subtract this from your TDEE. The remaining calories can come from fats or additional carbohydrates/protein if desired but not necessary.

Plan your meal frequency and Timing - Step 3

To optimise your protein intake, divide up your protein intake into 20-30g portions across 3 - 6 meals/day. If you are using supplements be sure to take these either before or after exercise to maximise their benefits. To stay well hydrated, follow the guidelines in Chapters 3 & 4 to optimise fluid retention and replenish loses.

Step 4 - Preparing for game day

Experiment with meal timing, frequency, and type in the days leading up to and day of training as a practice run for any competitions. This is very individualised so it will require some trial and error. Keeping a food diary of any side effects or effects on training are worth noting down to highlight what foods or practices you may want to avoid on game day. This is also a good time to experiment with carb and fat loading if you are an endurance-based athlete. If you are a strength/power-based athlete then this is of less benefit but can still help optimise glycogen stores before game day so it may be worth a try.

Include some flexibility and plan for special events - Step 5

You don't need perfect diet adherence to be a world-class athlete. Following a well-balanced, nutrient-dense diet that is 80 - 90% of your total caloric intake allows you to enjoy less healthier options the remaining 10 - 20% of your caloric intake. It can be easy to become obsessive over counting your macros and "eating clean" but this can lead to some unhealthy relationships with food. Therefore, include some flexibility, enjoy the occasional drink or take-away, just keep an eye on your weekly TDEE target and you'll be fine. The upside of exercise is you need to eat more so take advantage (in moderation of course).

Example Balanced/Varied Diet

Goals: 2,000 Calories/Day (14,000 Calories/Week), 75g Protein/Day, 2.0 Litres of Water/Day

	Day 1	Day 2	Day 3 (Fasting)
Breakfast	**Salmon, Eggs, & Avocado** (Poached Eggs, Smoked Salmon, Avocado, Flaxseed, Sourdough Toast) 400 ml of Water	**Overnight Oats** (Oats, Milk, Chia Seeds, Banana, Almond Butter) 400 ml of Water	**Just Water** (400 ml of Water)
Snack	**Greek Yoghurt w/Fruit & Nuts** (0% Greek Yoghurt, Maple Syrup, Blueberries, Crushed Mixed Nuts) 400 ml of Water	**Biltong** (South African Dried Beef & Game) 400 ml of Water	**Just Water** (400 ml of Water)
Lunch	**Prawn, Courgette & Pea Risotto** (Arborio Rice, Garlic, Spring Onions, Chicken Stock, Peas, Courgette, Mature Cheddar Cheese, Prawns) 400 ml of Water	**Rueben Sandwich** (Corned Beef, Sauerkraut, Blue Cheese, Thousand Island Sauce, Rye Bread) 400 ml of Water	**Just Water** (400 ml of Water)
Snack	**Just Water** (400 ml of Water)	**Carrot Sticks w/Hummus** (Sliced Carrots, Hummus Dip) 400 ml of Water	**Just Water** (400 ml of Water)
Dinner	**Moroccan Lamb Tagine** (Lamb, Onion, Garlic, Tomatoes, Sultanas, Almonds, Dries Apricots, Dates, Lamb Stock, Cayenne, Paprika, Ground Ginger, Turmeric, Cinnamon, Argan Oil, Honey, Coriander, Parsley, Couscous) 400 ml of Water	**Seafood Tagliatelle** (Salmon, Cod, Haddock, Prawns, Mussels, Milk, Bay Leaves, Butter, Garlic, Shallots, Leek, Plain Flour, Double Cream, Cayenne Pepper, Parsley, White Wine) 400 ml of Water	**Chicken & Mushroom Stroganoff** (Chicken Thighs, Brown Rice, Parsley, Chestnut Mushrooms, Garlic, Red Onion, Red Wine Vinegar, Smoked Paprika, Olive Oil, Lemon, Spinach, Greek Yoghurt) 400 ml of Water
Snack			**Spicy Mixed Nuts** (Cashews, Almonds, Walnuts, Brazil Nuts, Butter, Worcestershire Sauce, Paprika, Cayenne, Chilli, Cumin)

Day 4 (Meat-Free)	Day 5	Day 6	Day 7 (Treat)
Scrambled Tofu (Tofu, Turmeric, Black Pepper, Spinach, Mushrooms, Rye Bread)	**American Style Pancakes** (Oats, Banana, Eggs, Baking Powder, Salt, Cinnamon, Protein Powder, Ground Flax Seed)	**Coffee & Pastry** (Tall Cafe Latte, Almond Croissant)	**Toast w/Spread & Jam** (Multi-seeded Bread, Stanol Spread, Strawberry Jam)
400 ml of Water	400 ml of Water	400 ml of Water	400 ml of Water
Trail Mix (Mixed Nuts & Seeds)	**Cinnamon Cookies** (Oats, Cinnamon, Ginger, Coconut Oil, Honey)	**Just Water** (400 ml of Water)	**Just Water** (400 ml of Water)
400 ml of Water	400 ml of Water		
Lentil & Sweet Potato Soup (Sweet Potato, Red Onion, Cumin Seeds, Coriander, Garlic, Red Chilli, Red Lentils, Vegetable Stock, Coconut Milk, Lemon, Olive Oil)	**Sushi** (Nori, Rice Wine Vinegar, Mirin, Soy Sauce, Sushi Rice, Tuna, Sesame Seeds, Wasabi, Cucumber, Red Pepper, Shrimp Tails)	**Chicken Salad Ciabatta** (Watercress, Spinach, Rocket, Mayonnaise, Chicken, Red Onion, Ciabatta, Cucumber, Radish)	**Huel** (2 Scoops of Vanilla Black Edition Huel)
400 ml of Water	400 ml of Water	400 ml of Water	400 ml of Water
Roasted Chickpeas (Chickpeas, Mixed Spices)	**Fruit Salad** (Watermelon, Grapes, Pineapple, Mango, Cherries)	**Just Water** (400 ml of Water)	**Just Water** (400 ml of Water)
400 ml of Water	400 ml of Water		
Bean Chilli (White Onion, Carrots, Garlic, Tomatoes, Kidney Beans, Black Beans, Jalapeños, Bulgar Wheat, Coriander, Chilli Powder, Cumin, Black Pepper, Salt, Olive Oil)	**Mushroom Tacos** (Portobello Mushrooms, Bell Peppers, Onion, Garlic, Olive Oil, Paprika, Cum, Chipotle, Corn Tortillas, Greek Yoghurt, Avocado, Jalapeño, Mint, Black Beans, Cherry Tomatoes, Feta)	**Pepperoni Pizza** (4 Slices / Half a Medium Pizza)	**Five Guys Burger & Fries** Cheeseburger Little Cajun Fries Diet Coke
400 ml of Water	400 ml of Water	400 ml of Water	400 ml of Water
Protein Shake (Pea + Rice Blend Protein)			

INDEX

Q

R

S

We Want Your Feedback!

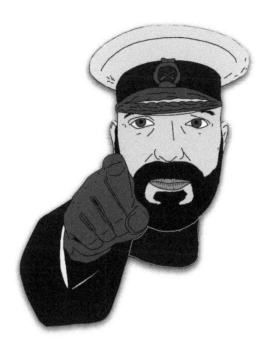

Did you enjoy this book? Did you find it helpful? Were there areas you think could be improved? Would you recommend it to a friend? We really want to know, so please consider leaving your feedback on Amazon, Waterstones, or at
www.eatmoveperform.com/books/emp-volume-1

You can also follow us on **Instagram**, **Facebook**, **YouTube**, and **Twitter** at @EatMovePerform and tag us with your pictures of you reading the book and we'll re-post our favourites.

@EatMovePerform
#EatMovePerform

Lightning Source UK Ltd.
Milton Keynes UK
UKHW052154130920
369756UK00003B/30